The Wholistic Menopause Handbook

Merging Hormone Therapy with Natural remedies

by
Well-Being Publishing

To You,

Thank you

Table of Contents

Introduction 2

Chapter 1: Understanding Menopause 3

Chapter 2: The Hormone Therapy Debate 11

Chapter 3: Nutrition for Menopause................................. 17

Chapter 4: The Power of Physical Activity......................... 24

Chapter 6: Managing Stress and Sleep 30

Chapter 7: Alternative Therapies and Approaches 36

Chapter 8: Sexual Health and Menopause......................... 43

Chapter 9: Holistic Skin and Hair Care 49

Chapter 10: Building a Supportive Environment............... 55

Chapter 11: Integrating Hormone Therapy with Natural
Remedies... 61

Chapter 12: The Role of Mindset in Menopause............... 67

Chapter 13: Preparing for Post-Menopause 73

Conclusion 78

Appendix A: Appendix.. 80

The Wholistic Menopause Handbook: Merging Hormone Therapy with Natural Remedies

Welcome to your journey through a milestone that's as natural as the dawn—menopause. As we embark on this path together, it's vital to embrace the idea that managing the shift in your body's rhythm can be as multifaceted and unique as you are. Think of the wholeness of your life—your nurturing spirit, your vibrant mind, and your energetic body; menopause touches them all, and this handbook is your ally, guiding you to synergize hormone therapy with the earth's bountiful, natural remedies. Traditions have long celebrated natural modalities, and modern science offers us hormone therapy advances. By intertwining these worlds, we'll craft a tapestry of wellness personalized for your body's needs. Menopause isn't the end of youth, it's the beginning of wisdom, and this chapter is your map to navigating through its nuances with grace and strength, using all the tools at your disposal for a balanced, joyous transition.

Introduction

Welcome to a space where your journey through menopause is honored and supported. As you navigate these transformative years, it's normal to feel a sublime mixture of empowerment and confusion. Menopause, a natural phase in the mosaic of womanhood, can be a time of profound change, and you shouldn't have to walk this path alone. This book is your trusted companion aimed at merging the contemporary wisdom of hormone therapy with the timeless benefits of natural remedies for a holistic approach to your well-being.

Within these pages, we embrace the multifaceted nature of menopause. We're not just talking hot flashes and hormone levels; we're delving into the emotional waves and the physical transitions that each tell a story unique to you. Think of this as your personal guide to decoding the messages your body sends and finding strategies that resonate with your lifestyle. From the food you savor to the movement that energizes you, and the rest that restores you, every chapter cultivates an understanding of how interconnected our bodily systems are and how they can be attuned during this stage of life.

Confronting the menopause experience head-on may seem like a daunting expedition, but imagine the empowerment that comes from harnessing knowledge and tools to illuminate your path. The goal here is to look beyond the traditional framework of menopause management and explore how you can tailor a comprehensive strategy that aligns with your values and vision of health. Let's set out together to create a balanced, joy-filled transition that's as natural and affirming as the dawn of a new day.

Chapter 1:
Understanding Menopause

As we close the first chapter on blending the modern wonders of hormone therapy with the age-old wisdom of natural remedies, let's pivot to truly grasp what menopause is all about. Imagine menopause as a profound transition, not just in your body, but in your very essence. Here we're talking about the reality behind the 'change of life,' demystifying the physiological metamorphosis that sounds so clinical yet feels incredibly personal. You're not just losing your period; you're gaining a new perspective on what health means post-fertility. We'll walk through the range of symptoms you might encounter, from the infamous hot flashes to the subtler shifts, acknowledging that while some experiences are universal, your menopause will be as unique as you are. And let's not sideline the emotional rollercoaster; those feelings of loss, confusion, or sometimes relief, they're all part of your journey. It's a tale of transformation, where the emotional landscape shifts as dramatically as the hormonal one. Here, we dive in, embrace, and truly understand menopause, wrapping our arms around its complexities and the self-knowledge that blooms from this pivotal time in life.

Defining Menopause and Its Symptoms

Menopause isn't just a phase; it's a significant transition, one that comes with a unique blend of physiological changes and symptoms that can catch even the strongest woman a tad off guard. It signals the end of the reproductive era when the monthly menstrual cycles take a bow, typically after twelve consecutive months sans period. We're talking about a time when estrogen and progesterone, those once-vibrant dance partners, start to slow their tempo, causing ripples that can be felt from hot flashes to mood swings. It's as personal as a fingerprint—while some may slight notice changes, others might face a torrent of waves, navigating through night sweats, sleep disruptions, and those moments of searching for words that dance just out of reach. Rest assured, the journey through menopause is a shared one, and while it might seem daunting, there's a spectrum of strategies to ease these tumultuous tides, combining the wisdom of hormone therapy with the harmony of natural remedies that can be tailored just for you. So let's lace up, embrace this transition with arms wide open, and transform these challenges into stepping stones for a vibrant, health-filled future.

The Physiology of Menopause isn't just a wave goodbye to your monthly cycle; it's a complex biological orchestra with your hormones at center stage. Imagine this: your ovaries have been your reliable hormone distributors for years, churning out estrogen and progesterone in a finely-tuned rhythm. As menopause approaches, this rhythm starts to change its beat – and not so subtly. It's like a dance floor where the music becomes unpredictable, causing quite the stir in the ways your body has grown used to moving.

Let's talk specifics. The dropping levels of estrogen, the hormone that's had your back since puberty, stirring the pot during your menstrual cycles and keeping your reproductive system in check, now decides to take a step back. And as estrogen levels decrease, so do progesterone levels, causing an array of physiological changes. Your body is incredibly savvy, and although it can feel like it's throwing you curveballs, it's actually readjusting to this new normal. Take hot flashes, for instance, those unexpected waves of warmth that can make you feel like you're in your own personal summer. They're your body's response to the hormonal shifts, more specifically the change in how your body regulates temperature.

It's not all heat waves and mood swings, though. This transition can stir up changes in your metabolism too, sometimes leading to weight gain. Plus, as estrogen takes a backseat, the risk of osteoporosis sneaks up because it's this very hormone that's been helping keep your bones dense and strong. And let's not forget the cardiovascular system, which also got some love from estrogen over the years. It's why staying heart-healthy becomes even more crucial during this time.

In the midst of these shifts, it's your moment to champion self-awareness and self-care. It's not about fighting against the current; it's about learning to surf the waves. Every body is different, so symptoms and experiences of menopause can vary significantly from one woman to another. How phenomenal is it that you can tailor your journey through menopause, equipped with knowledge and an array of strategies, embracing both modern medicine and time-honored natural remedies to find what works best for you?

Understanding the physiology of menopause is empowering. It's a time to recalibrate, to nurture your body through these changes. With each woman's experience being unique, the dialog between medical advice and holistic approaches becomes even more valuable. Have faith in this natural transition because, while it may seem tumultuous, it's a phase every woman navigates. And you've got this extraordinary capability to manage, adapt, and flourish, transforming challenge into opportunity. It's your body, embracing a renaissance, and you're the masterful artist at the helm.

Common Symptoms and Variations When diving into the sea of changes menopause brings, it's essential to recognize the shimmering facets of each symptom and its variations. Menopause is your unique journey, much like a snowflake, no two experiences are exactly the same. Hot flashes might be the talk of the town, yet they're just the tip of the iceberg. They can manifest as a sudden warmth spreading through your upper body or as a full-blown heat wave that makes you feel like you're on the equator. Some women might notice them more at night, disrupting sleep, while others deal with them throughout the day.

Irritability and mood swings often tag along with these temperature tussles. Picture your emotions as a pendulum, swinging unpredictably. One moment you might feel on top of the world, and the next, you're plunged into annoyance over the smallest things. These mood variations can strain relationships, but they can also offer a moment of insight into your needs and desires during this transformation.

Then there's the unpredictable menstrual cycle—it might shorten, lengthen, or take a solo trip without notice. Light spotting can turn into torrential rain, and this unpredictability might have you carrying a 'just-in-case' kit wherever you go. Sexual desire can also wane or surge, turning your intimate life into an unexpected adventure. The vaginal dryness that often comes into play here doesn't have to be a showstopper—with natural lubricants and open communication, you can choreograph a new sensual dance.

While these are some of the common headliners, don't overlook subtle signs like thinning hair, less elastic skin, or the bewildering sensation of crawling skin. Take a holistic view of these symptoms. They're not just nuisances; they're signals from your body, whispering or sometimes shouting for attention. Paying heed to these messages by adjusting your lifestyle, diet, and stress management strategies can make a profound difference in your well-being.

Ultimately, remember that variations are par for the course. A symptom that's a mere whisper for one woman can be a roar for another. Embrace the fact that your experience is uniquely tailored to you. With a spirit of exploration and the right arsenal of natural remedies complemented by hormone therapy, you can steer through the menopausal waves with grace and strength, ready to emerge with a renewed sense of self on the other side.

The Emotional Journey

Transitioning through menopause is nothing short of an emotional odyssey, an often bumpy ride marked by surges of feelings you may not have geared up for. It's as if your emotions decided to throw a spontaneous party, and you're the host without any prior planning. Let's unpack it together—understanding that the feelings aren't just rogue waves crashing over you, but a part of this natural process. It's common to feel like you're navigating a labyrinth, with mood swings and anxiety acting as shifting walls. Lean into the support of friends, speak freely with your practitioner about these mental somersaults, and carve out moments for self-reflection. Remember, this isn't just about getting through it, but growing through it; you're rediscovering and redefining your emotional landscape. Embrace the unpredictability with grace, and let's transform this journey into a path of empowerment and resilience.

Coping with Emotional Changes Life during menopause isn't just a series of physical shifts; the emotional rollercoaster can come with its fair share of ups and downs, too. While hormone therapy can ease some symptoms, emotions might still run high, and that's perfectly normal. Hormonal changes often influence mood and emotional well-being, so identifying strategies to cope with these changes is crucial for holistic health.

Firstly, understanding that mood swings, irritability, or bouts of sadness are all common companions to the menopausal transition can be a relief. You're not alone, and you're not at fault for these emotional fluctuations. A solid strategy involves embracing a balanced diet and regular physical activity—both of which can stabilize mood and improve overall well-being. However, don't dismiss the importance of adequate rest. Sleep disturbances are common during menopause, and they can exacerbate emotional instability. A focus on improving sleep hygiene can indirectly enhance your emotional resilience.

Mindfulness practices can also be a sanctuary for emotional health. Techniques like meditation, deep breathing exercises, or journaling provide an outlet for stress and help manage anxiety. Integrating these practices into your daily routine can create a buffer against the emotional undercurrents of menopause. And they're not just soothing—they can increase self-awareness, empowering you with the knowledge of what triggers your emotions and how best to respond to them.

Sometimes, though, the best soothing comes from solidarity. Establishing a reliable support system—family, friends, support groups, or a therapist—can provide the comfort and understanding you might be seeking. Sharing your experiences can normalize them, lessen feelings of isolation, and provide varying perspectives on coping. Don't underestimate the power of a good heart-to-heart or the occasional shared laughter; these are invaluable for emotional well-being.

Finally, if necessary, don't hesitate to reach out to a healthcare professional. Hormonal shifts can sometimes lead to more severe emotional health issues, such as depression or anxiety disorders, which may require professional support. There's strength in seeking help, and a tailored approach might include therapy, medication, or a combination of treatments that respect your journey through menopause. Remember, taking care of your emotional health is just as important as addressing the physical; both are intertwined on the path to holistic wellness.

Support Networks and Communication As we navigate the rythmns and cross-currents of menopause, the strength of our community and the clarity of our communication are lifelines. They uphold us in challenging moments and magnify our joy in times of triumph. So let's dive in with our hearts open, shall we?

Building strong support networks isn't just about having folks to lean on when times get tough; it's about fostering connections that are rooted in understanding and mutual nurturing. Whether this network comprises family, friends, fellow menopause navigators, or a support group, the essence lies in cultivating relationships that provide not just an ear for listening, but a voice for sharing and empathizing. Consider leveraging social platforms or joining online forums where many other women are sharing their menopause journeys. There's something incredibly empowering about knowing you're not alone in this, and these networks can turn into an invaluable resource for tips, recommendations, and shared experiences.

Now, about that other key piece—communication—it starts with you. Your ability to articulate your needs and experiences directly impacts the quality of support you receive. This means having open, honest conversations with loved ones and healthcare providers alike. Yes, menopause can sometimes feel like a taboo subject, but it's through dialogue that we demystify and destigmatize. When speaking with doctors or holistic health practitioners, be candid about your symptoms, your worries, and your goals for therapy and natural practices. A two-way street, this transparency fosters a collaboration that tailors treatments to your specific, holistic needs. It is essential to speak your truth—it's not just beneficial, it's necessary for your wellbeing.

While we're on the subject, let's not ignore the powerful act of communicating with ourselves through journaling or simply taking time to check in with our inner selves. Self-reflection not only helps us process our thoughts and emotions, it also contributes to our self-awareness, leading to clearer conversations with others. Journal prompts and symptom trackers (like the ones found in Appendix B) can be useful tools in this respect, helping to keep track of your experiences in a way that can later be articulated to others.

Lastly, remember that support and communication are dynamic—just like this journey you're on. They grow, they evolve, and they adapt. This can mean joining new groups, finding additional resources, or even moving on from relationships that no longer serve your progression. It's about flowing with the currents, not against them. In this dance of give and take, you'll find a harmony that not only supports you through menopause but enriches your life well beyond it. So, as you step forward, let these twin pillars of networks and communication chart a course that is enlightened, empowered, and ever progressing toward whole-hearted health.

Chapter 2:
The Hormone Therapy Debate

As we transition from understanding the what and why of menopause, let's wade into the waters of one of the most contentious topics that can't help but stir emotions: hormone therapy. Now, the concept isn't new and for generations, it's been at the heart of heated discussions. But let's face it, when you're hot-flashing more than you're hash-tagging, what you need is clarity. At its core, hormone therapy is about replenishing what your body once created naturally and that can sound pretty enticing. But it's a bit like navigating a maze – there are twists, turns, and it's easy to feel lost. So we're going to journey through this maze together, peeling back the layers of history, and pinpointing the benefits alongside the risks. It's more than facts and figures; it's about listening to your body and striking that sweet balance where you feel like you again. Stay tuned, because you're the boss here, and making an informed choice is your superpower.

Historical Use of Hormone Therapy

Imagine a journey back in time, when menopause wasn't something whispered about behind closed doors, but a mysterious change that countless women endured without much of a road map. It was the dawn of hormone therapy (HT), a time when medical professionals began viewing menopause not just as a phase, but a condition to be treated. It's essential to honor this narrative because it paved the way to today's nuanced conversation around menopause and wellness.

Our tale of hormone therapy begins in the 1940s and 1950s, when it was introduced as a revolutionary approach to alleviate menopausal symptoms. Initially, it was like a magic elixir for women, offering relief from hot flashes, night sweats, and other challenging symptoms. It can't be overstated how this science of synthesizing hormones changed lives. Women, who might have felt they were losing a part of themselves, found a new lease on life as hormone therapy promised to restore their youthful vigor and wellbeing.

By the 1960s and 1970s, hormone therapy gained even more popularity, cementing its place as a mainstay treatment. It was the heyday of HT, with the narrative suggesting that menopause was an estrogen-deficiency disease and HT the cure-all. Women were encouraged to take hormones long-term, not just for symptomatic relief but for purported benefits on skin, bone health, and overall vitality.

However, let's press pause and fast forward to the early 2000s, when studies like the Women's Health Initiative sent shockwaves through the world of hormone therapy, linking long-term use to an increased risk of breast cancer, heart disease, and strokes. It was a wake-up call, prompting women and doctors alike to rethink the blanket prescription of hormone therapy. The relationship between women and their hormones needed to be re-evaluated, with a spotlight on personal health histories, risks, and a more discerning approach to treatment.

So, here we are in the present day, with a more sophisticated understanding of menopause and hormone therapy. It's no longer about one-size-fits-all solutions; it's about tailoring treatments to individual needs, weighing risks and benefits, and often combining HT with natural remedies for a holistic approach. The historical narrative of hormone therapy isn't just background noise—it's a launching pad for informed decisions and empowered health choices as you navigate this transition. And remember, you've got resources aplenty to chart a course that's right for you and your unique journey through menopause.

Benefits and Risks of Hormone Therapy

Navigating the menopause transition can sometimes feel like you're trying to solve a puzzle with pieces that don't quite fit. One piece of that puzzle for many is hormone therapy, offering a beacon of relief for symptoms that can knock you sideways. Imagine regaining control, with less hot flashes and improved sleep, thanks to these medical advances. Your mood swings might not swing so wildly, and your bones can hold onto their strength a little tighter, shining a light on hormone therapy's potential to alleviate a range of bothersome menopausal symptoms. Yet, we can't ignore the whisperings of caution, with studies hinting at increased risks for some conditions like heart disease and breast cancer, especially with long-term use. Every woman's journey is as unique as a fingerprint; it's essential to keep that individuality in the forefront of our minds when considering hormone therapy. In this sanctuary of sisterhood, understanding the balance of benefits and risks is crucial—think of it as constructing a personalized roadmap for your wellness adventure, where informed choices about your body will light the way. Empowering yourself with knowledge will help you move forward, emboldened by the wisdom of your own experience combined with the medical insights that can support your menopause journey.

Weighing the Evidence Now, let's navigate through the sea of information regarding hormone therapy with the meticulousness of a seasoned sailor. As with any voyage, our direction must be informed by the stars, not by the waves that challenge us. In the case of hormone therapy, those stars are the studies, data, and findings that have emerged over years of exploration in women's health. Balancing hormones during menopause can be complex, and there's a plethora of research that both supports and questions the use of hormone therapy. It's key to sift through this with a critical eye, discerning what is most relevant to your unique situation.

Understanding the difference between correlation and causation in studies is as essential as distinguishing between a lighthouse and a star. Some reports show a relationship between hormone therapy and certain health risks or benefits, but this does not always mean one causes the other. Looking at large-scale, long-term research – like the landmark Women's Health Initiative study – can help clear the fog. Still, keep in mind that newer evidence and ongoing research often cast new light, advocating for a personalized approach to hormone therapy that considers individual risks, genetics, and lifestyle factors.

Diving into the pile of evidence, let's consider the perspectives of various experts and organizations. Evaluating their guidelines provides a balanced view of the potential advantages and limitations of hormone therapy. Equally important is to recognize the influence of non-medical factors – like diet, stress levels, and physical activity – in managing menopause symptoms. These lifestyle components work alongside hormone therapy, potentially enhancing benefits and reducing the need for higher hormone doses.

It's crucial to listen to your own body's signals as well. While research provides the map, your body's response offers the compass for adjusting your course. Some women find that hormone therapy works miracles in alleviating hot flashes, night sweats, and mood swings. Others may experience side effects or prefer to address symptoms with natural remedies before, or in conjunction with, hormone therapy. Honoring your personal health history and current well-being is fundamental in weighing the evidence for or against hormone therapy. This means regular check-ups, open communication with your healthcare provider, and introspection are all integral aspects of this process.

Lastly, let's blend wisdom with a sprinkle of patience. Decisions around hormone therapy don't have to be made overnight. Allow yourself the time to reflect on the information, consult with trusted medical professionals, and consider alternative remedies that align with your philosophy and lifestyle. The interplay of natural approaches, from herbal supplements to stress-reduction techniques, can provide a robust scaffold for your menopause strategy. In this journey, remember that you're the captain; stay informed, be adaptable, and keep your wellbeing as your true north.

Personalizing Your Decision

As you navigate the complexities of menopause and weigh the balance of hormone therapy with natural remedies, it's crucial to remember that this journey is deeply personal. Every woman experiences menopause differently, and the 'right' approach is the one that resonates with your unique body, lifestyle, and values. That's why, in this space, we're going to focus on tailoring your decisions to fit you, not just following a one-size-fits-all prescription. Your voice, your body's response, and your instinctual leanings are paramount in crafting a strategy that brings relief and vitality.

Consider your current symptoms—hot flashes may be your nemesis while another may find mood swings more disruptive. Exploring the range of natural remedies alongside hormone therapy can be a bit like having your gardening toolkit—sure, the spade is essential, but sometimes you need the finesse of the pruning shears. Do the legwork, get to know the tools at your disposal, and don't be afraid to reach out to healthcare professionals who respect your inclination towards a holistic approach and are eager to support you in your exploration.

While evidence stacks up on every side of the hormone therapy debate, only you can truly gauge how a particular treatment makes you feel. Are you more energetic, more 'yourself'? Or are you noticing side effects that dim the glow of the benefits? Remember, this isn't just science—it's your life and well-being at stake. Fostering open communication with your care provider allows for adjustments that better align with your evolving needs and preferences. It's a partnership where your well-being is the objective.

Diet and exercise are also essential considerations in this grand equation. Whole foods that are friends to hormonal balance could be foundational, as would a routine of exercises that invigorate rather than deplete. We'll dive into the specifics in the chapters ahead, but for now, remember: what you eat and how you move offer powerful complements to any hormonal treatment you undertake.

Ultimately, adopting a mindset that is both informed and intuitive is key to navigating this transition. The latest study or trend may provide valuable insights, but it's through listening and responding to your own experience with care and compassion that you'll find your path. Your menopause is yours alone—embrace the freedom to shape it into an experience that truly supports and uplifts you.

Chapter 3:
Nutrition for Menopause

Transitioning seamlessly from the hormone therapy debate, it's time we sink our teeth into the juicy topic of nutrition during menopause. It's not just about calming hot flashes or countering mood swings; think of food as your intimate ally, filling the role of comforter, healer, and balance-restorer all on one plate. Imagine: the joy of savoring a crunchy kale salad drenched in olive oil, not just for its vibrant flavors, but for the healing cascade it releases within you—this is the art of menopause nutrition. You're not just eating; you're replenishing and harmonizing your body's erratic symphony of hormones with every bite. Picking the right nutrients isn't just science; it's a personal journey, a discovery of the profound impact that food has not only on your physical well-being but on your holistic menopausal voyage.

Dietary Changes for Hormonal Balance

Embarking on the menopause journey can feel like you're adjusting to a new rhythm of life, full of nuances that weren't there before. One tune you can definitely set yourself to is that of dietary harmony. Food is a pivotal factor when it comes to balancing those temperamental hormones, and tweaking your diet might just strike the right chord. With a few considered changes, it's possible to help your body navigate the ebb and flow of hormone levels with grace and vigor.

Let's wade into the waters of phytoestrogens – these plant-based compounds mimic the effects of estrogen in the body, soothing the sometimes drastic dip in your natural levels. Tofu, tempeh, flaxseeds, and various other soy products are your new best friends. They're not only potential hormone helpers; they're also packed with protein and can help keep your heart in tip-top shape. But like any relationship, moderation is key; after all, you want a balanced ensemble, not a one-woman show.

Then, there's fiber – it's like your gut's diligent housekeeper, ensuring that everything runs just right. High-fiber foods help regulate blood sugar levels, manage weight, and keep your digestive system performing encores. Let's not forget its role in binding to excess hormones and whisking them away. Fruits, veggies, whole grains, and beans can help orchestrate this symphony of gut health and hormonal balance. Imagine your gut as an audience appreciative of a good performance, and you'll want to give it the best show every day.

Now, if your body were an instrument, omega-3s would be the maestro's wand, directing the show to reduce inflammation and possibly even the frequency of hot flashes. Fatty fish like salmon, mackerel, and sardines, plus chia seeds and walnuts, are exuberant in these essential fats. They're ready to take the lead in your journey toward hormonal equilibrium. You'll not only feel better, but you'll also be giving a standing ovation to your heart and brain health.

Lastly, let's cast a light on the supporting act of healthy fats. We're not talking about the stage hogs, the saturated fats – nope, we're spotlighting the understudies; the monounsaturated and polyunsaturated fats found in olive oil, avocados, nuts, and seeds. They aren't just filling in; these fats help with the absorption of vitamins and the production of hormones, ensuring the main performance — your well-being — is flawless. This is a supporting cast that you definitely want backing you every step of the way.

So, while there are no hard and fast rules about diet and menopause – every body dances to its beat, after all – leaning into these dietary changes can help manage menopausal symptoms. It's a symphony of small, mindful choices that, together, create a harmonious transition through one of life's natural intermissions. The interplay of food and hormones is complex, but much like understanding a difficult piece of music, once you grasp the essentials, you'll be playing like a seasoned maestro in no time.

Key Nutrients and Supplements

Transitioning through menopause, your body's nutritional needs take center stage. Imagine your body as a beautifully intricate system, requiring the right kind of fuel to ensure all gears run smoothly, especially when hormone levels fluctuate. Certain key nutrients and supplements can be game-changers here. Calcium and vitamin D are pivotal for maintaining bone density, warding off the specter of osteoporosis. Omega-3s aren't just good for the heart; they also combat inflammation, potentially easing those pesky joint aches. Let's not forget about the B vitamins and magnesium — they're like the unsung heroes for energy metabolism and mood regulation. And for those nights when sleep seems elusive, and hot flashes come knocking, phytoestrogens from sources like flaxseed and evening primrose oil, alongside a good dose of vitamin E, can be your secret arsenal for comfort. Tread this journey with a stash of these essential nutrients and your body will thank you, with resilience and vitality that keep you thriving through menopause and beyond.

Vitamins and Minerals to Focus On As you weave through the rich tapestry of menopause, understanding that your body's nutritional needs evolve is your very own wand of empowerment. As your hormonal landscape shifts, certain vitamins and minerals become crucial allies. Let's illuminate some key nutrients that deserve a VIP seat at your table, serving as not just guests but co-hosts to support you through this transformative chapter.

First up is calcium, and for good reason. You see, estrogen plays a pivotal role in maintaining bone density, and as estrogen levels ebb, your bones might whisper (or shout) for a little extra love. Calcium steps into this spotlight magnificently, but it can't perform solo. Vitamin D, its steadfast partner, enhances calcium absorption, reinforcing bone strength and helping steer you clear of osteoporosis' unwelcome embrace. Embracing foods rich in these nutrients, or considering supplements, along with your healthcare provider's nod, can be a smart move.

Next, let's chat about magnesium. This maestro of minerals not only dances in harmony with calcium for bone health but eases into the role of a pacifier, potentially calming those pesky hot flashes and supporting your earnest quest for sound sleep. It's a mineral that doesn't scream for attention but subtly supports over 300 bodily reactions, including mood regulation—something you might find particularly soothing when riding the emotional rollercoaster commonly associated with menopause.

Then there's the B-vitamin ensemble, particularly B12, B6, and folate. As energy synthesis and cognitive function become top-of-mind concerns, these nutrients are akin to a backing band that keeps the rhythm of your life upbeat. B-vitamins can impact everything from energy levels to brain fog, lending a hand in keeping your mental clarity as sharp as your wit. And don't overlook their contribution to heart health; they have a part in keeping homocysteine levels, an amino acid linked to heart disease, in check.

Lastly, let's not forget about antioxidants like vitamins C and E. They're the guardians against oxidative stress, associated with a host of age-related ailments. Vitamin C bolsters your immune system, while vitamin E is believed to have a positive influence on skin health and possibly, hot flash frequency. Incorporating a myriad of colorful fruits and vegetables into your diet can create a vibrant palette from which these antioxidants can paint a robust picture of health.

Aligning with these nutrient powerhouses can be a delightful exploration. Each one brings something unique to your holistic health canvas. Remember, while shopping the aisles for these nutrients or browsing for supplements, it's about creating a collaborative symphony with your body's needs. Always consult with a healthcare professional for tailored advice because your journey is as personal as the intricate tapestry woven by your experiences, and you're the artist holding the brush.

Herbs and Phytoestrogens As we delve into the role of nature's bounty in easing the transitions of menopause, it's essential to cast light on the powerful allies found in herbs and phytoestrogens for balancing hormones naturally. Embracing these botanical gifts can open doors to newfound balance and well-being during a phase of life that's both challenging and transformative.

Herbs have been the cornerstone of traditional medicine for centuries, cherished for their ability to heal and harmonize the body. When it comes to menopause, certain herbs have risen in popularity owing to their reputed benefits in mitigating symptoms such as hot flashes, night sweats, and mood swings. These include but are not limited to black cohosh, red clover, dong quai, and even the humble licorice root. Each herb offers unique properties that can complement the body's changing landscape during menopause.

Arming yourself with knowledge about these natural remedies lets you navigate your menopausal journey with a sense of empowerment. For instance, black cohosh, with its long history of use among Indigenous peoples, has been researched for its potential to mimic estrogen in the body, which might help to curb hot flashes and improve mood. It speaks to the heart of finding solace and support in nature's apothecary.

Then there's the intriguing world of phytoestrogens, naturally occurring plant compounds that function similarly to estrogen within the human body. Foods rich in phytoestrogens, such as soy, flaxseeds, and sesame seeds, might offer a more gentle approach to hormone balance. These compounds can bind to estrogen receptors and may help alleviate some of the hormonal fluctuations that lead to menopausal symptoms.

Integrating these phytoestrogens into your daily diet can be as simple as sprinkling ground flaxseed on your morning oatmeal or enjoying a refreshing glass of soy milk. It's these small, consistent acts of self-care that weave together a tapestry of holistic health. Creating wholesome meals not only fuels your body but also becomes an act of nourishing your soul.

Yet, while enthusiasm for these natural therapies is well-founded, it's crucial to approach them with a balanced perspective. Not every herb or phytoestrogen source is right for every woman, and their effectiveness can vary based on individual factors. Consulting with a healthcare provider or a herbal medicine expert can guide you to make choices that are safe and fit your unique health profile.

It's also of utmost importance to consider the quality and sources of these natural remedies. The market is vast and not all products are created equal; seeking out organic, non-GMO, and sustainably harvested herbs will ensure you're nurturing your body with the purest ingredients. Plus, supporting ethical and environmentally-conscious companies aligns with a holistic lifestyle that honors both personal health and the planet.

Dosage and interactions are another vital aspect that should not be overlooked. Some herbs and phytoestrogens may interact with medications, and certain conditions may contraindicate their use. Therefore, a personalized approach that's fine-tuned to your needs—not just following the latest trends—is key to effectively using these natural wonders.

Remember, the journey through menopause is as much about the soul as it is about the body. Embracing herbs and phytoestrogens isn't just about seeking relief from symptoms; it's also an invitation to reconnect with the natural world and to rediscover a sense of wholeness.

As you weave these natural components into your larger menopause strategy, you'll be stepping into a dance with nature, one that carries the rhythm of your own body's wisdom. Honor that rhythm, listen to its cues, and allow yourself the grace to adapt and experiment. Combining the modern aspects of healthcare with the enduring wisdom of herbal remedies can illuminate the path to vitality and equilibrium during menopause.

Chapter 4:
The Power of Physical Activity

As we turn the page from exploring the role of nutrition in menopause, it's time to lace up our sneakers and delve into Chapter 5: The Power of Physical Activity. It's no secret that our bodies evolve with time, and during menopause, it can feel like we're in the middle of a seismic shift. But don't fret! Engaging in regular physical activity can be a game-changer. It's not just about weight control; it's about taking the reins of your health during this transformative time. From reducing hot flashes and bolstering your mood to improving sleep quality, and even sharpening your mind – the benefits are as vast as the horizon. And it's not about hitting the gym hard or running marathons unless that's your jam. It's about finding joy in movement, listening to your body, and cultivating a routine that's sustainable, revitalizing, and most importantly, personalized to suit your unique journey. So, let's get moving, discover exercises that lift you up, explore the direct link between an active lifestyle and symptom relief, and empower you to enjoy this natural, potent elixir for holistic menopausal health.

Exercise for Symptom Relief

Let's talk about the magic of movement and how it can be a game-changer for navigating the symphony of menopause symptoms. Exercise isn't just about keeping fit; it's a powerful ally in soothing some of those pesky menopausal challenges. From hot flashes to mood swings, it turns out breaking a sweat on purpose can actually help chill out those spontaneous sweat sessions. Research is in your corner, too, showing that women who incorporate regular physical activity into their lives experience fewer and milder symptoms. So, let's lace up those sneakers and get moving towards relief.

Picture this: you're in the middle of a hot flash, and the last thing you feel like doing is a workout. Totally understandable. But, there's good news. Moderate exercise has been shown to help reduce the frequency and intensity of hot flashes. Think of it like this - exercise helps regulate your internal thermostat. It's not an instant fix, but over time, you'll likely notice a difference. Plus, activities like yoga and pilates? They're fabulous for stretching out the tension, calming your mind, and, yes, even helping with those temperature tantrums.

Mood swings got you feeling like you're on an emotional roller coaster? Exercise releases endorphins, those feel-good hormones that boost your mood and act like natural painkillers. And it doesn't have to be high intensity to be effective. A brisk walk in the park or a calming swim can do wonders for your state of mind, helping to combat anxiety and depression. It's about finding what lifts your spirits and gets your body grooving. It's okay to start small – the key is consistency, and the benefits for your mood will unfold with time.

Sleep woes are another common refrain during menopause. The sleep-exercise relationship is a two-way street. Regular physical activity can help you fall asleep faster and deepen your sleep. Just be mindful of timing; try to wrap up any vigorous exercise a couple of hours before bedtime, so you're winding down when you hit the pillow. Gentle, restorative practices like tai chi or a tranquil evening walk can serve as a perfect prelude to a night of restorative slumber. Imagine resting more peacefully and waking up feeling energized – exercise can help escort you there.

Lastly, let's touch base on the muscle and bone support exercise offers. As estrogen takes a bow, it can leave a gap in the spotlight where bone density and muscle mass used to shine. Strength training, resistance exercises, or even just carrying groceries can help fill that gap, maintaining strength and supporting bone health. Start with weights that challenge you but don't strain, and progressively get stronger over time. Balance and flexibility exercises also aid in preventing falls, an important consideration as we reach wiser years.

Empower yourself through the menopausal transition with a physical activity that resonates with you, your needs, and your lifestyle. It's a proactive step you can take at your own pace, in your own space, and it can make all the difference. Remember, every little bit counts, and your body and mind will thank you for it. Let the power of physical activity be the unsung hero in your menopause journey!

Finding Your Ideal Workout

Let's dive into the curative waves of physical activity, honing in on that sweet spot where exertion meets exhilaration. It's all about discovering the workout regimen that makes your heart sing while easing those pesky menopausal discomforts. Whether it's the endorphin rush from a brisk walk or the muscle-awakening stretch of yoga, finding the right exercise for you is like unlocking a secret garden of vitality amidst the fluctuating landscape of menopause. Let's be clear: it's not about attaining perfection or competing with your past self—pursue what feels good, provides relief, and fills you with joy. As you sift through the variety of fitness avenues, remember, this journey is intrinsically yours, and your ideal workout is there, waiting for you to lace up your sneakers or roll out your mat. So, let's get moving, let's be kind to our bodies, and let's embrace each stride and pose with open arms, because your path to hormonal harmony can indeed be paved with the steps of your favorite dance routine or the calm resilience of tai chi.

Cardiovascular Health during menopause becomes a noteworthy topic of discussion, not just a checkmark on your list of health concerns. The heart is quite the trooper, steadfastly beating through every stage of life, but menopause can throw a few curveballs its way. Estrogen, the hormone taking a bow during this phase, plays a rather protective role in vascular health. So, when levels start to dwindle, keeping your heart health in check becomes super important. Let's dive into why staying active can be a game-changer for your ticker.

First off, regular cardiovascular exercise is the star player in maintaining a strong heart. It's like a gym session for your heart, which needs to stay in shape just like any other muscle. Kick-starting your routine with a brisk walk, progressing to a jog or finding joy in a dance class not only uplifts your spirits but keeps the blood flowing smoothly. It decreases the risk of developing high blood pressure, a common menopausal bonus, and helps regulate weight. Remember, the 'use it or lose it' principle applies here – keeping active ensures your heart stays in top-notch condition.

Now, you might wonder about the intensity and frequency of such activities. Well, the answer lies in finding a balance that works for your life. Aim for at least 150 minutes of moderate aerobic activity or 75 minutes of vigorous activity spread throughout the week – maybe a combo of both. It's not about running marathons (unless that's your jam); it's about consistency and enjoyment. Whether it's a nature hike, swimming, or a cycle around the park, select an activity that doesn't feel like a chore. This is your journey, and treating your heart right should feel rewarding.

Of course, we can't ignore the importance of diet in cardiovascular health. Those leafy greens, whole grains, and omega-3 rich foods you've heard about? They're not just good; they're great for heart health. Combine a well-rounded diet with your exercise routine to pack a one-two punch against heart disease. But it's not just about adding the good stuff; it's also wise to cut back on excess salt, sugar, and unhealthy fats that can contribute to heart woes.

Lastly, let's not forget the role stress plays in cardiovascular health. That pesky stress can increase blood pressure and, over time, wear out the heart. So, while you focus on keeping your body moving, also embrace practices that calm your mind and soothe your soul. Yoga, deep breathing, or meditation can be fabulous companions on this journey, contributing to reduced stress and better heart health.

Wrapping it up, keeping your heart healthy during menopause is all about making mindful choices every day. The art of living well is an intricate dance between activity, nutrition, and peace of mind. So keep lacing up those sneakers, choosing the salad (yes, with avocado), and taking those moments to breathe deeply. Your heart will thank you for it, and you'll be setting the stage for a vibrant, healthy life post-menopause.

Strength and Flexibility - these are pillars of physical wellness that tend to wane as we navigate the shifting sands of menopause. Maintaining muscle strength and supple joints is not only about looking good, it's crucial for keeping our independence and vitality as we age. Think about it; every day, your body performs a symphony of moves - reaching, bending, lifting - and with compromised strength or flexibility, that symphony starts hitting sour notes, ones that can limit your quality of life.

So let's talk strength training. It's not just for the bodybuilders among us. Adding a few sessions a week can serve as a keystone habit that brings a myriad of benefits. Strength training increases lean muscle mass, which in turn, revs up your metabolism. This can be particularly helpful as menopause may slow down your metabolic rate. Now, we're not just talking dumbbells and machines; bodyweight exercises, resistance bands, and even daily activities like carrying groceries or gardening all count towards building strength. The goal here isn't to lift the heaviest weights, but to challenge your muscles consistently and safely.

And then there's flexibility - the art of moving effortlessly and without pain. Yoga or Pilates can be fantastic for this, but so can simple daily stretch routines. Flexibility training helps alleviate stiffness and improves range of motion, reducing the likelihood of injury and enabling you to perform everyday tasks with ease. Just a few minutes a day devoted to stretching can make a significant difference. And who knows, those few minutes might become your daily haven of tranquility and a chance to reconnect with your changing body.

Of course, the fear of injury or the misconception that "I'm not the gym type" can hold many back from embracing these activities. What's vital to understand is that strength and flexibility workouts should be tailored to your individual level and gradually increased as your abilities develop. Always listen to your body, and if you can, seek guidance from a fitness professional who understands the nuances of menopause and can help create a program that's just right for you.

Remember, you're not trying to compete with anyone else or turn back the clock to your twenties. This is about crafting a strong, flexible you, for future-you. Strength and flexibility training are powerful allies in your toolkit for a vibrant menopausal transition. They'll not only help manage some symptoms of menopause but also set you up for a healthier, more active post-menopausal life. Embrace the challenge with kindness and patience, and you'll be amazed at what your body can achieve.

Chapter 6:
Managing Stress and Sleep

Transitioning from an energizing discussion of physical activity in the last chapter, we smoothly segue into an equally crucial aspect of menopausal life—managing stress and embracing restorative sleep. We all know the frustration of lying awake, our minds a whirlwind of to-dos and what-ifs. Add to that menopausal hormone fluctuations, and calm slumber might seem like a distant dream. But here's our collective embarkment on harnessing stress and unfolding the secrets of serene sleep. With practical strategies tailored for the complexities of menopause, we'll explore how to transform our bedrooms into sanctuaries of peace and our minds into allies for tranquility. It's time to elevate our nightly routine from a toss-and-turn saga to a peaceful rejuvenation—a powerful reclamation of control in a time of change. Composure and quality sleep aren't just luxuries; they're the bedrock of a holistic approach to thriving through menopause.

Mindfulness and Relaxation Techniques

In our journey through managing stress, we arrive at a serene stop—you guessed it—mindfulness and relaxation techniques. For many women navigating the occasional stormy seas of menopause, finding peace and serenity can be as vital as a lighthouse guiding a ship to shore. Now, mindfulness—what's the buzz about? Imagine it as a gentle anchor, keeping you rooted in the present, even when hot flashes and mood swings feel like they're pulling you out to sea. It's about acknowledging these moments without judgment. And relaxation? It's the counterbalance to stress, a gift that you can give yourself daily.

Let's dive into a few methods that can help buoy you up. Starting with deep breathing exercises: they're simple, yet powerful. When you're feeling engulfed by anxiety or a wave of hormones, pause and take a deep breath. Inhale slowly, filling your lungs, and exhale even more slowly. Picture your stress floating away on the breeze—it's a reset button for your nervous system. Integrating these breathing techniques into your daily regimen isn't just refreshing; it's scientifically shown to encourage a state of calm.

But perhaps breathing alone won't do the trick, so let's explore another haven—guided imagery. This technique harnesses the power of your imagination to whisk you away to a peaceful place, a personal sanctuary where menopause's hot flushes and night sweats don't reign. Whether it's a sunlit beach with the rolling waves as your soundtrack or a silent forest with a carpet of soft, green moss, these mental vacations can significantly reduce stress levels. Paint these scenes in your mind, complete with sensory details, and watch as your stress melts away.

Of course, let's not forget about one of the most celebrated practices today—yoga. With its graceful blend of movement and breath, yoga does wonders for the mind and body. It stretches away physical tension while the meditative aspects can smooth out mental creases. And the best thing? Yoga can be as gentle or as challenging as you need, making it a perfectly adaptable friend during menopause. Add in a splash of meditation after your practice, sitting quietly or perhaps chanting a soothing mantra, and you've got yourself a potent cocktail for inner peace.

Finally, let's tap into progressive muscle relaxation—another jewel in the crown of de-stressing techniques. It works by tensing and then releasing each muscle group in the body, inviting you to dance along the fine line between strain and relief. It's almost like giving a silent nod to each part of your body, acknowledging the hard work it does and granting it permission to relax. This dance can be particularly effective before bedtime, paving the way to a restful night's sleep—a treasure trove we'll be exploring next.

In wrapping up, consider these techniques your trusty toolkit, ready whenever menopause tries to rock the boat. They're more than just strategies; they're proof of your commitment to your well-being. With each mindful breath, each visualization, and every purposeful stretch, you're building resilience against stress. And never forget—you're not alone on this voyage. Millions of women are navigating these same waters. So here's to mastering the art of mindfulness and relaxation. It's about taking the reins and becoming the serene captain of your own menopausal journey.

Sleep Hygiene for Better Rest

As dusk arrives and the world quiets down, it's time to prioritize your sanctuary of slumber. Sleep hygiene isn't just about having a comfy bed, it's an entire routine that preps you for optimal rest. Think about a nightly unwind; perhaps a cup of herbal tea and a good book to signal the body it's time to ease into dreamland. Keep gadgets to a bare minimum in the bedroom – their glow can meddle with your natural sleep rhythm. Regular sleep and wake times go a long way, as consistency is king for catching those Z's. The temperature, too, is a key player - keep it cool, creating an ideal nest that supports your bodies' need to drop its core temperature for sleep. Remember, your bedroom should be a cave of quiet and dark, a retreat that tells every cell in your body, "Hey, we're safe; let's recharge." So let's nudge those pesky worries off the pillow and embrace the night with open arms – your menopausal journey deserves that restful anchor.

Creating a Restful Environment As we turn the page on managing stress and sleep, let's focus our attention on nestling into the serenity a well-crafted sleep space can provide. Mouthfuls of advice tell us that sleep is paramount, but here, we're going to transform those words into a sanctuary where rest isn't just a possibility—it's a nightly reality. Imagine your bedroom; now, let's turn it into a haven that encourages the ultimate slumber, especially during the unpredictable nights menopause tends to bring.

First, consider the palette of your room. Colors can significantly influence our mood and emotions. Soft, muted tones often lend themselves to a calming atmosphere. Think pastels, earthy hues, or just the sophisticated simplicity of creams and whites. These shades can act like a gentle whisper, telling your body it's time to wind down. And it's not just about what you see—texture plays a comforting role, too. Outfit your bed with sheets that hug you back; natural fibers like cotton or bamboo breathe well and caress the skin, inviting you to drift away into dreamland.

Your senses are powerful, and each can be appeased to promote better sleep. Let's talk about the soundtrack of your slumber. The soft hum of a white noise machine can blanket any disruptive sounds, cradling you in consistency. Maybe you're more soothed by the lull of nature's symphony—a babbling brook or the gentle call of night creatures. There are countless apps and gadgets to fill your room with these tranquil auditory hugs. And don't forget the olfactory magic - a dab of lavender oil or the sweet whisper of chamomile from a diffuser can do wonders for relaxing the mind and preparing you for sleep.

Now, the right ambiance is only half the battle—the other is thwarting the interruptions. Make your bedroom an electronic-free zone if you can. Yes, that means parting, even momentarily, with your beloved devices. The blue light emitted is like a stimulant for your brain when it should be sinking into sleep. Also, finding the right temperature is key; everyone's different, but a slightly cooler room often makes for better sleep. Experiment until you find your sweet spot, perhaps with breathable pajamas or even a weighted blanket for that hugged sensation.

Lastly, rituals can have a tremendous impact. A routine signals to your body that it's time to shut down. This can be as simple as a cup of herbal tea while reading a book, a few gentle stretches or deep-breathing exercises, or jotting down a few thoughts to clear your mind. Remember, finding rest can be a fluid thing; what works now may need tweaking later. Be kind to yourself, stay patient, and allow your restful environment to evolve with your needs through this journey of menopause. Your body—and your mind—will thank you for every night of restorative sleep you gift them.

Natural Sleep Aids

A good night's sleep can seem elusive during menopause, but it's more than just a mere luxury. Sleep is indispensable, an ally in your journey through this phase. Simply put, restful sleep can be a game-changer, positively influencing not just your mood, but also the way your body handles menopausal transitions.

There are numerous natural sleep aids that you can incorporate into your nightly routine to foster better sleep. A tried and true favorite is a warm cup of chamomile tea. Chamomile has been used for centuries to promote relaxation and sleep, thanks to an antioxidant called apigenin that binds to certain receptors in your brain, reducing insomnia, or the chronic inability to sleep.

Another remedy to consider is Valerian root, often referred to as "nature's Valium". Many women find it to be a helpful sleep aid during menopause. Its extract has been shown to improve the quality of sleep and the speed of falling asleep — without the 'hangover' effect some experience with sleep medications.

Melatonin supplements can also be beneficial. Melatonin is a hormone naturally produced by the body that regulates sleep. Its levels fluctuate throughout the day, peaking at night to promote restful sleep. During menopause, however, these levels can decrease, influencing the quality of sleep. Taking a melatonin supplement can help to re-balance these levels, promoting better sleep patterns. But remember, it's important to approach supplements cautiously and consult with your healthcare provider before starting a new regimen.

Finally, consider implementing mind-body practices into your bedtime routine. Techniques such as progressive muscle relaxation (PMR), deep-breathing exercises, and guided imagery can promote relaxation and pave the way to a better night's sleep. They can help quiet the mind, release physical tension, and tap into a deep sense of calm and well-being. After all, you're not just sleeping; you're nurturing your body and embracing the stillness that nighttime brings. When it comes to menopause, that peaceful, restorative nighttime quiet can be a powerful ally. Seize it, embrace it, and sleep tight!

Chapter 7:
Alternative Therapies and Approaches

After delving into the power of sleep and stress management in the previous chapter, let's embrace the vibrancy of alternative therapies that might just be the missing piece in your menopause management mosaic. Picture a world beyond the conventional; acupuncture's fine needles rebalancing your energy flow, easing hot flashes and inviting calmness. Imagine the subtle power of homeopathy, and suppose naturopathy's natural remedies could complement the balance you seek. This chapter isn't about choosing sides—it's about opening doors. It's about validating the whispers of intuition that guide you toward a more harmonious state of well-being. As you journey through menopause, let's explore these pathways with open hearts and minds, understanding that each woman's map to wellness is uniquely her own, and within the diversity of these approaches, there might just be a therapy that resonates with you, helping to restore the symphony of your body's natural rhythms.

Acupuncture and Acupressure

As we navigate through the shifting tides of menopause, let's explore two compelling stars in the vast sky of holistic health: acupuncture and acupressure. These ancient practices are rooted in Traditional Chinese Medicine and are believed to channel healing by manipulating the body's vital energy, or qi. For many women stepping through the threshold of menopause, these therapies can be a wellspring of relief, tapping into the body's own capacity to restore balance and alleviate symptoms.

Acupuncture involves the insertion of fine needles into specific points on the body. It's not about just poking around hoping for a quick fix—it's a deeply considered art, backed by centuries of refinement. You might be curious whether those tiny needles can really cool down those hot flashes, ease those mysterious aches or soothe the storm-tossed sea of hormonal mood swings. Well, many women find that they do. It's thought that acupuncture needles may influence the body's hormonal balance, providing a natural nudge towards equilibrium without the need for synthetic interventions.

On the flip side, acupressure is acupuncture's needle-free cousin. Here, the healing power is at your fingertips—literally. By applying pressure to specific points, you can engage the same energetic pathways, but in a gentler fashion. It's a self-empowering approach that you can learn and use anywhere, be it your office chair or the comfort of your living room. For those middle-of-the-night awakenings or sudden onset of symptoms when a professional isn't on hand, acupressure may become your go-to self-help tool for instant relief.

While the needles and pressure points tackle the physical, there's also an undeniable tranquility that accompanies these practices. The calm environment of an acupuncturist's clinic or the meditative focus required for self-acupressure can invite a state of deep relaxation. This serenity itself can be a balm for the sleep disruptions and stress that often accompany menopause. It's not just about tending to the body's invisible energy lines—it's also about carving out a moment of peace in your bustling day-to-day life. Women in the throes of menopausal turbulence sometimes discover that their sessions are oases of calm in an otherwise hectic world.

However, always approach these therapies with a curious yet cautious mind. Investigate practitioners thoroughly to ensure they are certified and experienced, especially with menopausal concerns. Even though acupuncture and acupressure are generally considered safe, every woman's journey is unique—what sings harmony for one may not resonate with another. It's important to listen to your body's symphony and adapt accordingly. If you decide to embark on this path, know that these age-old practices might interweave beautifully with other strategies, contributing to a holistic tapestry of menopause management.

Homeopathy and Naturopathy

As you navigate the complex landscape of menopause, you might be drawn to the gentle embrace of homeopathy and naturopathy, realms of healing that complement the rhythm of your body's natural transitions. Imagine unlocking the secrets within nature's own medicine cabinet—homeopathy works on the principle of 'like cures like,' where tiny doses of natural substances aim to coax your body into a self-healing mode, striving for a unique harmony that whispers wellness back into balance. And then, walk along the nurturing path of naturopathy—a bouquet of botanicals, nutrition, and lifestyle modifications tailored just for you, with the goal of igniting your body's intrinsic healing potential. These therapies are not one-size-fits-all; they're like a dance choreographed to the music of your individual needs and symptoms. They beckon you to be an active participant in your health, to explore and discover natural alternatives that resonate with your personal journey through menopause. As you consider blending these age-old practices with modern treatments, it's an empowering step towards holistic harmony in your life's symphony.

The Role of Holistic Practitioners in menopause management is a beacon of individualized care in a sea of generalized medical advice. These practitioners come from a wide spectrum of disciplines, including naturopathy, homeopathy, acupuncture, and others. They share a common ground in that they look at the person as a whole, rather than focusing solely on the symptoms or the menopause itself. Working with a holistic practitioner means you're acknowledging that menopause isn't just a hormonal change—it's a life transition that touches every facet of your being.

For many women, the guidance of a holistic practitioner can demystify the crossroads between conventional hormone therapy and the multitude of natural remedies available. Holistic practitioners typically spend more time getting to know you—their approach goes beyond just your medical history. They're interested in your stress levels, dietary habits, exercise patterns, emotional health, and spiritual wellbeing. This information helps to create a tailored action plan that not only navigates the physical symptoms you're experiencing but also enriches your overall quality of life during this transformative time.

The beauty of holistic care is its capacity for integration and complementation. While some may have reservations about blending natural remedies with hormone therapy, holistic practitioners often thrive in finding the balance that works specifically for your body and lifestyle. They're your partners in steering through the sometimes overwhelming wave of herbal supplements, dietary adjustments, and lifestyle changes, pinpointing which will likely work in synergy with any hormone treatments you're considering or currently using.

Engaging with holistic practitioners also paves the way for empowerment through education. Learning how to listen to your body's signals and understanding the deeper reasons behind specific treatment recommendations can be incredibly freeing. Rather than passively following a prescription, you're actively participating in your health journey. The goal isn't just to manage menopause; it's to emerge on the other side feeling knowledgeable and in control of your wellness path.

Finally, a notable aspect of holistic care is its emphasis on prevention and maintenance. By working on underlying health patterns now, you're setting up sturdier foundations for post-menopause health. Holistic practitioners can provide insights into long-term strategies for maintaining bone density, heart health, mental acuity, and more. As you collaborate with these professionals, remember that your journey through menopause is unique, and you deserve a care approach that's as multifaceted and dynamic as you are.

Evaluating Alternative Treatments You've been journeying through the nuances of menopause, exploring everything from hormone therapy to the power of diet and exercise. Now, let's venture into the realm of alternative treatments, which can be exciting yet also overwhelming with its myriad of options. It can be hard to distinguish between what truly promotes well-being and what is merely anecdotal. So, how do you evaluate alternative treatments and find what resonates with your unique experience of menopause?

Firstly, research is your ally. It's not just about finding a quick fix to alleviate hot flashes or mood swings; it's about understanding how different therapies interact with your body. Scientific studies are invaluable, though the research on some alternative treatments might not be as extensive as conventional medicine. Weigh documented benefits against any potential risks, and look for studies that are peer-reviewed and have solid methodology.

Secondly, don't underestimate the power of personal testimonials but take them with a grain of salt. Hearing firsthand accounts of how a treatment has worked wonders for others may be compelling, yet it's crucial to remember that every body is different. What works for one person may not work for another. Understanding this can save you from frustration if a highly praised treatment doesn't yield the same results for you.

Thirdly, tap into professional insight. Consult with healthcare providers, especially those who specialize in women's health and holistic medicine. They can provide an informed perspective on whether a certain herb or acupuncture could beneficially integrate with your current health plan. They'll also help you monitor your health to ensure any alternative treatments don't interfere with any medications or therapies you're currently undergoing.

And it's not just about the physical symptoms. The emotional transitions during menopause can be just as taxing. Seek out therapies that address your emotional and psychological well-being, such as meditation, yoga or tai chi. These practices have been shown to reduce stress and improve mental health, which often correlates with a reduction in physical symptoms as well.

Consider the source of the alternative treatment as well. Is the provider certified? Are the herbs or supplements you're considering from a reputable source? Unfortunately, the market is flooded with false claims and low-quality products, so always ensure you're choosing treatments based on quality and credibility.

Dosage and duration are also crucial. Some treatments might have a cumulative effect, requiring consistent application before noticeable benefits occur. On the other hand, if you're not seeing results or you're experiencing adverse effects, it's important to reevaluate whether to continue.

Financial aspects can't be ignored; while health is invaluable, it's also important to consider the cost of alternative treatments, many of which are not covered by insurance. Analyze if the costs are sustainable over the long term, especially if it takes time to see benefits.

Moreover, integration is key. If you've found a natural remedy or practice that you believe in, think about how it will fit into the broader picture of your health. Alternative treatments should complement your lifestyle and medical care, not replace them. An adept balance between traditional and alternative approaches has the potential to provide the most comprehensive relief.

Lastly, remember the journey of menopause is deeply personal. What resonates with you, feels right, and aligns with your values is key. While you might gather information, opinions, and advice, at the end of the day, the choices you make should empower you and support your journey in a way that feels authentic. Embrace the process of exploring, trying new things, and adjusting as you go. Each step is a learning opportunity that contributes to your wellness tapestry.

Armed with these evaluation strategies, you're better prepared to navigate the sea of alternative treatments with confidence. Your well-being is a tapestry woven from many threads – hormone therapy, diet, exercise, and now, alternative treatments. As each woman's tapestry is unique, your approach to integrating these treatments will be just as individualized. Listen to your body, stay informed, and trust that you're on the right path towards a holistic health strategy that truly resonates with you during menopause.

Chapter 8:
Sexual Health and Menopause

Embarking on menopause can feel like setting sail into a mysterious sea where the waves of sexual health seem to shift unpredictably. It's completely natural to notice changes in your libido and find that what once ignited your passion has evolved. But don't worry, you're not adrift. Embracing this new stage means redefining what intimacy looks like for you and your partner, and recognizing that communication is your compass in these uncharted waters. This chapter is your guide to navigating those sometimes turbulent seas with confidence. We'll delve into natural ways to maintain comfort and pleasure, from exploring personal lubricants that harmonize with your body to embracing comfort measures that enhance connection. Let's set sail on this journey of rediscovery, where sexual wellness continues to be an integral, vibrant part of your life's tapestry. Remember, menopause might be a transition, but it can also be a time of profound intimacy and growth.

Navigating Changes in Libido

Embracing the ebb and flow of sexual desire can be one of the more challenging nuances as you journey through menopause. It's kind of like the tide – sometimes it's in, sometimes it's out, and it's influenced by a variety of elements. Understanding that shifts in libido are a normal part of this transition is crucial. While hormone fluctuations certainly play a big part, your overall health, stress levels, and emotional wellbeing are co-stars in this drama. Here you'll find solid ground to stand on when the waves of menopause try to knock you off balance.

It's worth exploring how hormone therapy might fit into your libido's narrative, but don't forget to look beyond it. It's just as important to consider natural remedies and lifestyle changes that can complement such treatments. Whether it's adapting your diet to include more phytoestrogens, finding the right exercise routine to invigorate your body, or using mindfulness to reconnect with your own sense of sexuality, there are numerous paths to explore. Each step you take can serve as a life raft, keeping you buoyant even when things seem adrift.

It's okay to feel perplexed or frustrated as you try to figure out what works best for you. The key is to listen to your body's rhythm and not to pressure yourself to adhere to past standards or expectations. This may be a time of experimentation and discovery – finding what kind of touch sparks joy for you now or which activities fuel your sense of intimacy. It's all about adapting and creating new ways to experience pleasure and connection, and these can evolve into a rejuvenated sense of self and confidence in your sexuality.

The dialogue around sexual wellbeing during menopause is often whispered, but let's turn up the volume. Engage in frank conversations with your healthcare provider about all the options, from lubricants to deal with vaginal dryness to ways to address the psychological components of desire. Support groups and forums can be great places to share experiences and receive emotional support, helping you remember you're not navigating these tides alone.

Remember, your libido isn't just about sex; it's about vitality and life force. Nurturing it during menopause can mean the rekindling of old flames or the sparking of new ones. This isn't just a time of loss; it's a time of transformation and potential growth. So, take it one step at a time, stay patient and open-minded, and let your journey of self-discovery unfold. The changes in libido are not just a hurdle to overcome but an opportunity to deepen your understanding of your body and desires.

Intimacy and Relationship Dynamics

As you navigate the rippling waves of menopause, the intimate shores of your relationship might seem a little more complex. Hormonal shifts can have a tidal pull on your desire and the very nature of physical connection. It's common, and totally okay, to notice changes in the way you experience intimacy—and it's important to recognize that this is a shared journey. You're not alone, and this phase can actually deepen the bonds of your relationship through open communication and understanding. Reinventing intimacy often means exploring new territories together, from the emotional to the sensual, and finding balance in your evolving desires. Think of it as an opportunity to rediscover each other and yourself. By approaching these shifts with a spirit of curiosity rather than anxiety, you create space for warmth and closeness to flourish anew in your partnership, despite menopause's changing tides.

Communicating with Your Partner

When the winds of menopause start to blow, they seldom breeze through without rustling some feathers in our intimate relationships. Let's face it: hormonal changes can have us feeling like we're riding an emotional rollercoaster, and this doesn't just affect us, it also affects those closest to us—especially our partners. Communication is the bridge that can keep you both on solid ground, even when everything else feels like it's shaking. Start by talking openly about what you're experiencing. It's okay to acknowledge that things are changing and that you might need a little extra patience, understanding, or even space at times. Remember, though, it's not just about what you say, but how you say it. Approach each conversation with honesty and kindness to foster a supportive dialogue.

Understanding is a two-way street; encourage your partner to share their feelings as well. Menopause might be your physiological journey, but it impacts the emotional landscape of your relationship. Ask them how they feel about the changes they're witnessing in you and your relationship. This isn't an easy talk to have, and you might not solve everything in one go, but opening up this channel of communication can relieve tension. Furthermore, as you navigate the waters of hormone therapy and natural remedies, invite your partner to learn with you. Share articles, book excerpts, or even attend a consultation together. Knowledge can empower both of you, making room for empathy and partnership in decision-making as you traverse this transformative phase together.

Your intimate life might also feel the ripples of menopause, and it's vital to communicate about this realm of your relationship with sensitivity and openness. If you're experiencing changes in libido or discomfort during intimacy, speak up rather than retreat in silence. Explore natural lubricants and comfort measures, and remember, intimacy comes in many forms—it's not solely about physical love but also about emotional connection. Cherish small gestures, delve into new realms of closeness, and be inventive. Working together as a team to maintain the bond you share is itself an act of love, one that can grow and deepen despite, and perhaps because of, the challenges menopause brings.

Natural Lubricants and Comfort Measures Venturing into the scenic landscapes of your sexual well-being during menopause can feel a bit like navigating uncharted waters—both exciting and, at times, a bit daunting due to changes in natural lubrication and comfort. Fortunately, Mother Nature provides an array of natural lubricants that can enhance intimacy without the side effects that some synthetic products might introduce. Let's explore some options that embrace the wisdom of the natural world while honoring the sacredness of your body's new rhythms.

Firstly, consider the wonders of water-based lubricants. These are a fantastic go-to for their purity and ease of use, and they're compatible with most contraceptives and toys. Aloe vera, revered for its soothing properties, headlines the ingredients list in many water-based formulas. This plant holds moisture like a sacred vow, offering relief not only externally but sometimes helping to alleviate internal dryness as well.

If a richer texture is what your body craves, oil-based lubricants could be the answer. Coconut oil, revered for its versatility, not only nourishes your kitchen creations but also brings a luxurious, tropical feel to your private moments. This natural emollient supports skin health while providing the necessary slick for a smoother experience. However, do remember that oil can degrade latex condoms, so be sure to consider alternatives if protection is a priority.

Itching for options that go beyond immediate relief? Hyaluronic acid and vitamin E supplements are the unsung heroes among natural comfort measures. They may not be the traditional route for addressing vaginal dryness, but their regenerative properties can be a boon for long-term tissue health. Incorporating these supplements could potentially contribute to natural lubrication over time and amplify your body's ability to maintain moisture.

Finally, don't forget the power of foreplay and patience. Menopause might have changed the pace at which your body responds, so taking the time for arousal to build can be both a form of self-care and a way to enhance natural lubrication. This mindful approach to intimacy can transform your experience, turning a potential challenge into a journey of rediscovery with your partner or during your solo explorations.

Remember, the path to comfort is as unique as you are. As you embrace this phase of life, keep an open mind and play with different natural options to find what feels best. With every tender touch and choice of lubricant or comfort measure, you're honoring the incredible journey that your body is on—recalibrating, renewing, and redefining what pleasure means in the context of menopause. Trust in nature's bounty and your own wise intuition to guide you through this exploration with grace and ease.

Chapter 9:
Holistic Skin and Hair Care

Moving on from sexual health, it's time to dive into the world of holistic skin and hair care - because, let's face it, these external aspects of our wellbeing often reflect what's going on inside our bodies during menopause. Fluctuating hormones can turn your skin and hair into unpredictable territories, with changes in texture and moisture levels. But there's good news: you can nurture them back to radiance with the right natural approach. The secret to glowing skin and luscious locks isn't locked away in expensive bottles; it's about understanding what your body's going through and how to support it with the kindness it deserves. Embrace nourishing routines that align with nature's wisdom, choose products that are friends to your body and the environment, and discover the joys and effectiveness of DIY treatments. This chapter isn't about vanity – it's about honoring your body through these powerful years of transformation and claiming the confidence you rightfully own.

Addressing Hormonal Impact on Skin and Hair

Navigating through menopause can feel like you're charting a new course through uncharted waters, especially when it comes to the changes in your skin and hair. The hormonal roller coaster can really throw your body's largest organ, the skin, and your once luscious locks, for a loop. Your skin might feel drier, less elastic, or perhaps it's suddenly prone to breakouts you thought you left behind in your teenage years. Your hair may thin out, or become more brittle and less voluminous. But here's a gentle reminder: These changes are a natural part of the menopausal transition and there are empowering ways to address them holistically.

Let's first understand that estrogen plays a significant role in maintaining skin hydration, elasticity, and hair health. As estrogen levels decline, you might witness your skin lose some of its youthful glow and plumpness due to decreased collagen production. This isn't merely cosmetic; your skin is a protective barrier and maintaining its health is vital. So, how do we nurture our skin from the inside out? Diet is key here. Emphasizing foods rich in omega-3 fatty acids, like flaxseeds and walnuts, and antioxidants found in fruits and veggies, can support skin health. Coupling good nutrition with gentle skincare practices paves the way for radiant skin through menopause and beyond.

When it comes to hair, the thinning you might be experiencing is also largely due to hormonal shifts. It's frustrating, we know, but there are steps you can take that don't involve harsh chemicals or invasive treatments. Think of scalp care as an extension of your skin care routine. Gentle, natural shampoos paired with regular scalp massages using essential oils like rosemary or lavender can stimulate circulation and potentially encourage hair growth. Also, be mindful of heat styling and harsh hair treatments that can further damage delicate strands during this sensitive time.

Beyond topical treatments and nutrition, don't underestimate the power of stress management and quality sleep. Stress can exacerbate skin issues and contribute to hair loss, while sleep is a time for the body to heal and rejuvenate. Incorporate mindfulness or relaxation techniques into your daily routine to help manage stress levels. And remember, sleep is not just quantity, but quality too. Create a restful sleep environment and consider natural sleep aids to help you get the rejuvenating rest your body craves.

Ultimately, while hormonal changes during menopause are inevitable, they don't have to dictate your skin and hair's health. Embracing a holistic approach that includes a balanced diet, proper skin and scalp care, stress relief, and restorative sleep, you can feel confident and in control during this natural life transition. Yes, your skin and hair may not be the same as they were in your twenties, but with attentive care, they can still be vibrant and reflect your inner health and vitality. Remember, you've got this!

Natural Skincare Routines

As we navigate through the tides of menopause, our skin begs for a touch of tenderness—and what's more nurturing than infusing natural elements into our skincare routines? Imagine your skin, a blooming garden that thrives on gentle, pure ingredients. Step away from harsh chemicals and let's embrace the wisdom of plant-based oils, rich in antioxidants, to bring back that supple youthfulness. In this chapter, we're handpicking nature's best to protect and rejuvenate your skin as it adapts to hormonal changes. Whether it's luscious coconut oil that caresses your skin into hydration, or the soothing caress of aloe vera, reducing redness and calming irritations, let's craft a regime that resonates with the very essence of Mother Earth. Through trial, joy, and maybe a little mess in the kitchen, whip up face masks and gentle cleansers that celebrate your natural beauty. And remember, every brushstroke on the canvas of your skin paints towards a masterpiece of self-love and radiance in these transformative years. Embrace this journey; let's pamper our skin with nature's touch and watch it flourish.

Choosing the Right Products In the sea of skincare products aimed at combating the signs of aging and hormonal changes, it feels overwhelming, doesn't it? To ensure efficacy and safety, especially during menopause, it's crucial to navigate these waters with care. Your skin, now more than ever, requires gentle, nourishing ingredients that understand the language of transformation your body speaks.

Choosing the right skin care products in menopause isn't just about vanity; it's about finding solace for skin that can feel as unpredictable as your hormone levels. Begin with a patch test to gauge sensitivity—your skin may react differently now than it did in years past. Opt for products with natural moisturizers like hyaluronic acid, which can help retain skin's dwindling moisture. Antioxidants like vitamins C and E are also your allies, protecting skin from free radicals and encouraging rejuvenation.

Likewise, be mindful of what isn't in your products. Parabens, sulfates, and fragrances can often do more harm than good, leading to irritation and discomfort. Seek simplicity in ingredients—less truly can be more. And don't underestimate the power of a great sunscreen. Regardless of the product, make 'spectrum' your favorite word, because UVA and UVB rays don't play favorites with age.

Don't forget, your scalp and hair face their own challenges during menopause. Products infused with natural oils, such as argan or coconut, can support hair strength and luster without weighing it down. Gentle, sulfate-free shampoos will clean without stripping essential oils, and don't overlook the potential scalp-soothing properties of tea tree oil. Remember, nurturing your hair starts with understanding its current needs, which can shift just as much as your hormones do.

Ultimately, navigating which products to embrace during this stage of life is about trial, attention, and adjustment. Start with what your skin and hair are telling you—they're the most honest critics you'll find. And while you're exploring the aisles, stay tuned into research and expert recommendations, but also trust your intuition. After all, embracing your holistic health during menopause also means listening to the wisdom of your body—it knows more than it gets credit for. Embrace this journey with tenderness and patience, and you'll find the harmony your skin and hair have been yearning for.

DIY Treatments and Remedies

After exploring the benefits of a well-rounded skincare routine, let's dive into the treasure trove of homemade concoctions that can add a dash of radiance to your skin and luster to your hair during menopause. Creating these remedies in the comfort of your own kitchen isn't just cost-effective; it's empowering. You have control over what you're putting on your body, and the natural ingredients can work wonders without the need for harsh chemicals. So, let's mix up some magic with ingredients likely already nestled in your pantry, ready to soothe, moisturize, and rejuvenate.

When it comes to hydration, your skin craves it, especially now. One of the simplest, yet profoundly effective treatments is a facial mask made from honey and avocado. Full of natural fats and moisture, avocado nourishes skin deeply, while honey, with its antibacterial properties, can give your complexion a clear and glowing boost. Combine it with a touch of yogurt, and you've got a gentle exfoliating mask that can help slough away dead skin cells and reveal the smooth, soft skin beneath.

Now let's talk about your locks. Hormonal changes can leave your hair feeling less than luscious, but a homemade hair mask can be your ally. A favorite involves massaging coconut oil with a bit of essential lavender oil into your scalp and hair. Not only does it smell heavenly, it helps combat dryness and can even promote relaxation—an added bonus when stress levels are high. Wrap your hair in a warm towel and let the oils work their magic before washing as usual. Your hair will thank you with shine and softness.

But DIY remedies aren't just about what you apply; it's about what you consume too. Infusing your water with skin-friendly ingredients like cucumber, lemon, or mint not only makes hydrating more enjoyable but also supplies your body with antioxidants. While we're in the realm of consumption, let's not forget about teas. Herbal teas like chamomile or red clover aren't just for sipping; they can double as soothing facial steams or toners, thanks to their anti-inflammatory properties.

Lastly, let's acknowledge the power of self-care rituals. These DIY treatments are more than skin-deep—they're a means to dedicate time to yourself, to nurture your body and soul in a season of change. And as you whisk and blend these natural remedies, remember that each ingredient is a dollop of self-love. Embrace this time with grace and find joy in the process, because taking care of yourself is a beautiful expression of self-respect and vitality.

Chapter 10:
Building a Supportive Environment

As you turn the page on the tactics of self-care and the importance of maintaining social ties, let's dive deeper into tailoring the world around you to support your body's profound evolution during menopause. It's about enveloping yourself in an atmosphere where positivity blooms, much like a garden perfectly suited for growth. Imagine crafting an oasis where every interaction and element genuinely nourishes your well-being—this isn't a spa day luxury, it's a fundamental right. This sanctuary extends beyond the confines of your home; it's woven into the fabric of your daily routines and circles of friendship. We'll explore how to cultivate your environment—realizing that the ground you walk on, the air you breathe, and the company you keep can either be a buffer against the tides of change or a booster rocket propelling you to new heights. Here, we put emphasis on the power of connection, the rejuvenating quality of laughter shared with friends, and creating spaces that resonate with comfort. By consciously curating your surroundings, you're not just adapting to change; you're inviting joy and resilience to hold firm ground in your life.

Social Connections and Activities

Transitioning through menopause can feel like you're navigating uncharted waters—often choppy and unpredictable. But here's a life raft for you: forging strong social ties and engaging in satisfying activities can anchor your days with joy and companionship. Consider this—friends truly are the lifelines that can pull us out of the isolating tides of menopause. Whether it's reconnecting with old pals over brunch, joining a book club, or even participating in a walking group, having conversations that go beyond hot flashes and hormone therapy can breathe fresh air into your life.

Some activities seem like they were tailor-made to nourish our spirit during times of change. Take a moment and think back to the hobbies you've set aside or new interests you've contemplated exploring. Now's the time to dive in! Ever wanted to paint, garden, or learn a new instrument? There's immense healing in the arts and creativity. Not only do these pursuits give a satisfying outlet for self-expression and stress relief, but community classes can also connect you to others who share your interests, fostering a sense of belonging and mutual support.

Volunteer work is another avenue that often gets overlooked. It's not just about giving back; it's a two-way street. You provide a service or help to someone in need, and in return, you find purpose and perspective. Engaging in your community can also expose you to a diversity of experiences and viewpoints, which can be incredibly enriching during this phase of your life. And let's not forget the power of just a good old-fashioned chat—sharing stories and laughter with someone can be wonderfully therapeutic.

Of course, navigating social circles during menopause might require setting some new boundaries. It's okay to take a step back from relationships that feel draining or unfulfilling. Cultivate an environment where you can thrive by seeking out positive, uplifting people who understand what you're going through. Look for menopause support groups, either locally or online, where you can discuss not only the challenges but also celebrate the triumphs. Where you can be heard, valued, and truly seen.

So, let's lace up those shoes, step out of our comfort zones, and connect. Embrace the plethora of activities that await you and the multitude of folks who are eager to journey alongside you. As you build your network, remember to savor these relationships and experiences; they can bring light during the days when you need it most. After all, it's the shared moments of humanity that often become the cushioning that softens life's edges.

Redefining Self-Care

In this transformative period of your life, self-care isn't just a luxury; it's a vital component of your well-being. The art of self-care is evolving, transcending the occasional bubble baths and facials to encompass activities that nourish you on a deeper level. Think of it as building a personal toolkit that can help you navigate the ebb and flow of menopause-related challenges. Whether it's carving out time for a reflective walk, feeding your body with wholesome, nutritious foods, or engaging in creative outlets that spark joy and stimulate your mind, each act of self-care is a step toward holistic health. These personal rituals are your secret superpower, offering respite and rejuvenation amidst the whirlwind of hormonal changes. And let's not forget, your self-care practices empower you to emerge stronger and more resilient, ready to take on the world with grace and vigor.

Establishing New Routines It's no secret that amidst the rush and tumble of life changes, especially during menopause, forging new patterns can provide a much-needed anchor. Routines are the scaffolding that can hold us steady when our bodies are sending us on a hormonal roller coaster ride. It's all about honing in on actions that serve your well-being, and repetition is your friend. Establishing new routines doesn't mean a complete overhaul—it is about integrating small but significant habits that nurture health on all fronts.

Now, let's talk about mornings. They can set the tone for the day ahead. While the temptation might be to hit the snooze button and burrow under the covers, consider starting with just ten minutes of stretching or meditative breathing. It's like sending a gentle but firm memo to your body: you're taking care of it. Over time, these ten minutes of focused self-care might just become a non-negotiable part of your day, a ritual that signifies that you're putting your health first—mentally and physically.

What we put into our bodies becomes even more crucial during this whirlwind time. Introducing a routine centered around nutrition could be pivotal. This doesn't mean you need to sacrifice flavor or joy in eating. It's the opposite, really. It's about creating a rhythm of nourishing your body with foods that can help balance hormones and boost energy levels. Picture this: weekly meal planning, involving colorful veggies, quality proteins, and maybe some experimental cooking with phytoestrogen-rich ingredients. It's as much about what's on your plate as it is about the ritual of preparation and enjoyment.

Don't forget that stillness can be as important as activity in our routines. Carving out time each day—perhaps before bed—to engage in quietude is a powerful routine to develop. Maybe it's journaling, perhaps it's reading or even dipping into a lavender-scented bath. Whatever the practice, let it be a time when you listen to what your body needs, a moment to decompress and prepare for restful sleep. Remember, routines that promote good sleep hygiene can be game-changers, especially when sleep disturbances are a common sidekick of menopause.

Last but certainly not least, think about your support system. Can your routine involve a weekly check-in with a good friend or a support group for women embarking on this same journey? These connections, consistent and nurturing, are invaluable. There's strength in the shared experience—knowing you're not alone can make all the difference. Building a routine that includes reaching out regularly ensures you stay grounded and connected, turning to one another for wisdom, comfort, and a healthy dose of laughter.

Ultimately, these new routines are more than just a schedule on a calendar. They are acts of self-respect, affirmations that your health and well-being are paramount. Change isn't just something to cope with; it's an opportunity to rebuild and renew. Your routines are the steps you climb, patiently, persistently, as you journey through menopause towards a space that is uniquely yours, where tranquility and vitality coexist. Embrace these practices with kindness to yourself, knowing that with each new day, you're nurturing not just a routine, but a new beginning.

Embracing Change - it's a phrase that often evokes a mix of apprehension and anticipation. As you journey through menopause, this concept becomes not just a suggestion but a necessity. Change is at the very core of menopause; your body is shifting, redefining normal every day. But let's not just endure this transformation, let's lean into it with grace and curiosity. Whether it's tweaking your diet to support hormonal balance, incorporating a new exercise routine, or simply adopting a new skincare regimen harmonious with your evolving needs – embracing change can be incredibly empowering.

It's human nature to hold onto the familiar, but the beauty of menopause is that it invites you to reassess, to realign your lifestyle with your body's current narrative. This could mean exploring relaxation techniques like mindfulness to not just alleviate stress but also to deeply understand the nature of your thoughts and emotions during this time. It might be daunting at first, but there's a certain thrill in discovering new paths to well-being that resonate with the person you're becoming.

Embracing change also extends to your social life and self-care routines. Perhaps it's time to nurture new friendships with those who are walking a similar path, or maybe it's about setting boundaries that allow you more time for rest and rejuvenation. Self-care is non-negotiable during menopause, and what that looks like for you right now could be very different from what it was a few years ago. Indulging in activities and practices that feed your soul and body is not coddling—it's essential maintenance for your holistic well-being.

Understanding that change can also manifest in your relationships, maintaining open lines of communication with your partners, friends, and family is key. Menopause can reshape intimacy and connection, making it important to express your needs and concerns. Natural lubricants and comfort measures for sexual health, as discussed later on, can be part of this dialogue. Change is not just within you; it's within the intricate web of your relationships, too.

Finally, a word on the mental reframe that embracing change requires. This isn't a farewell to your former self but an open-armed welcome to the multitude of possibilities ahead. It's about making peace with transitions and recognizing them as growth opportunities. Yes, there will be moments of resistance, but with each small step towards acceptance, you're building resilience and a profound sense of agency over your menopause experience. So let's celebrate every nuance of this chapter; after all, it's uniquely yours to shape.

Chapter 11:
Integrating Hormone Therapy with Natural Remedies

As we lace together the wisdom from hormone therapy and the gentle touch of nature, remember that the symphony of your body's needs sings its own unique tune. Imagine weaving strands of resilience with threads of tranquility as we explore how to harmonize hormone therapy with the gifts that earth's apothecary offers. It's like conducting an orchestra where every instrument has its place—pharmaceutical and plant-based remedies working in concert. As we embark on this chapter, let's unpack how to complement those science-backed treatments with herbal whispers and nutritional nudges. You'll find that alongside the structure of hormone treatments, there's a flow of natural remedies waiting to soothe, energize, and align with your body's rhythm. We're talking a tailored blend that respects your individual journey—because let's face it, no one knows your body like you do. With open ears and hearts, we'll sift through the possibilities, empowering you to make choices that resonate with your lifestyle and wellness goals. You've got this, and together, we'll find that balance that lets your spirit soar right through menopause.

Tailoring Treatments to Individual Needs

Embarking on the menopause journey is truly a personal adventure, and it's vital to remember that there's no one-size-fits-all approach to wellness. As we dive into the captivating world of combining hormone therapy with natural remedies, it's essential to shape each strategy to fit snugly to your unique needs and situation. After all, your body speaks a language as distinctive as your personality, and learning to interpret and respond to its signals is crucial to achieving balance and harmony during this transition.

When considering hormone therapy, it's critical to factor in your individual symptoms and their severity, medical history, and lifestyle. This is when a tightly-knit collaboration with your healthcare professional becomes invaluable. They can guide you through the options, whether it's a bioidentical hormone approach or a low-dose traditional regimen, and then you can sprinkle in the natural remedies that resonate with you. Maybe it's the calming embrace of yoga alongside a phytoestrogen-rich diet, or perhaps acupuncture sessions that complement your hormone patches. The canvas is yours to paint, and each brushstroke of personalization can lead to a masterpiece of relief and well-being.

Tuning into your body also means being attentive to how it evolves over time. Changes in how you feel and react to treatments are completely normal and expected. That's why adjustments to dosage, frequency, and types of therapy aren't just common; they're a sign you're in tune with your body's changing needs. As natural supplements or stress-reduction techniques become more or less effective, you'll navigate these adjustments with confidence and grace, knowing that with each small shift, you're optimizing your path to comfort and vitality.

In your toolkit of natural remedies, diversity is your ally. The synergy between various practices like mindful meditation, dietary adjustments, and the judicious use of supplements can work wonders. This integrative approach not only supports hormone therapy but empowers you to take proactive steps in managing menopause your way. Leverage the strength of this synergy, always keeping an eye on how your body and emotions respond, ensuring that both science and nature are working in your favor.

Last but definitely not least, it's about heeding the rhythms of your life and aligning your treatments accordingly. Small tweaks can make significant impacts. Maybe it's adjusting meal plans to better suit your energy levels or choosing restorative workouts that align with hormonal fluctuations. And as you listen and learn, share these insights with your health team, because this journey is a partnership. Together, you'll craft a menopause experience that's as unique as you are, weaving hormone treatments and natural remedies into a personal tapestry of wellness that supports you through menopause and beyond.

Monitoring and Adjusting Treatments

Embarking on the journey of hormone therapy while embracing natural remedies isn't about setting a course and sticking to it rigidly; it's about being in tune with your body and making changes when they're called for. As you continue to layer these strategies, it's essential to monitor your body's responses, from mood swings to hot flashes. Noticing subtle shifts can be the difference between feeling okay and feeling great. Be sure to keep a symptom diary—you'll find this can be an incredibly insightful tool, providing a clear picture of your progress and any patterns that emerge. Regular check-ins with your healthcare provider are key to ensuring your hormone levels are optimal, and these professionals can help adjust dosages or suggest new natural remedies based on your feedback. Remember, your body is unique, and so too should be your treatment plan. Sustained well-being during menopause is a dynamic dance, and you are the choreographer, beautifully synchronizing the rhythm of hormone therapy with the natural remedies that nourish and support you.

Setting Goals and Expectations As you navigate the intertwining pathways of hormone therapy and natural remedies for menopause, it's essential to establish clear goals and realistic expectations. Where are you heading on this journey, and what do you wish to achieve along the way? Make your goals as tangible as you can. Perhaps you want to mitigate hot flashes to the point where they're no longer disrupting your days or to improve your sleep quality. Each goal will become a stepping stone to your overall well-being.

Start this process by taking stock of your current situation. Which menopausal symptoms are affecting you most? What impacts your quality of life the hardest? It's important to prioritize. Let's say, if restless nights and mood swings top your list, then your initial goals might focus on establishing better sleep hygiene and finding stress-relief practices that resonate with you, all while considering how hormone therapy can contribute to these goals.

Setting expectations is equally vital. It's about recognizing the balance between optimism and patience. Changes won't happen overnight, and the road might have its bumps. Hormone levels and bodily responses are as unique as fingerprints; what works wonders for one may not for another. So, prepare yourself to be flexible and to track your progress. Adjustments may be necessary—switching up supplements, tweaking hormone dosages, or trying new relaxation techniques—as you learn what resonates with your body.

Collaborate with your healthcare providers to set these goals and calibrate your expectations. Remember, they're here to support you, listen to you, and help you navigate this multifaceted approach. Communication is key—don't hesitate to ask questions and share your concerns. They should know the details of your journey as it unfolds. This two-way street of information will guide them in helping you modify your strategy as needed for the best outcomes.

Lastly, set goals beyond symptom relief. Menopause, although challenging, is also a time to rediscover yourself and grow. Aim to strengthen your relationships, pick up new hobbies, or engage in community activities. Cultivate a mindset that embraces the changes and propels you toward a fulfilling and vibrant post-menopausal life. With well-defined goals and grounded expectations, you're setting yourself up for success in this holistic journey of health and self-discovery.

Staying Informed and Updated And now, let's take a stroll down the road of continuous learning. When it comes to integrating hormone therapy and natural remedies, you're in it for the long haul. Your body is unique, and so is your menopause journey. That's why staying informed and updated is not just a recommendation; it's a cornerstone of your wellness strategy. The medical field is always bustling with new research, and alternative health practices continue to evolve. So, consider this your gentle nudge to keep your curiosity alive and your knowledge fresh.

First up, let's talk about resources. Finding credible and up-to-date information might seem daunting, but here's a lifeline: medical journals, reputable health websites, and menopause-specific organizations are all excellent starting points. Tailor your research to suit your journey. Are you experiencing a new symptom? Has something in your lifestyle changed that might affect your menopause experience? Dive into the latest studies or connect with online forums and support groups where other women share their insights and experiences. Remember, the collective wisdom of those walking the same path can be an invaluable asset.

An equally important step is maintaining a solid relationship with your healthcare provider. The right practitioner will not only listen and validate your concerns but also stay abreast of current trends in hormone therapy and natural health. You'll want someone who can discuss the latest findings with you and collaborate on adjusting your treatment plan as needed. They should be a partner in your health journey—one who keeps the communication channels wide open and encourages you to ask questions and voice concerns.

Finding your rhythm with tracking your symptoms and responses to various treatments is also crucial. Keeping a detailed journal can help you see the patterns you might not notice day-to-day. Have you found certain dietary tweaks ease your hot flashes? Did a new yoga class bring a sense of wellbeing and relieve anxiety? Noting these observations provides hard data you can bring to your practitioner, making it easier to navigate the ever-expanding landscape of options and tailor your plan precisely.

Lastly, embrace flexibility in your path to wellness. Your body's needs may change as you move through different stages of menopause, and so might the information available to you. Give yourself permission to shift gears, try new approaches, and discard what no longer serves you. Your needs are not static, and neither should be your approach to staying informed. To thrive during menopause, keep your heart open to change, your mind keen for knowledge, and your spirit resilient against the waves of uncertainty. Know that the quest for balance is a profound journey of self-discovery and health empowerment.

Chapter 12:
The Role of Mindset in Menopause

Transcending the physical aspects of menopause requires a reshaping of our mental landscape. This chapter delves into the transformative power of a positive mindset, a potent ally in your journey. The way we frame our experiences with menopause can actively influence our body's response to them—creating a ripple effect that can either soothe or exacerbate symptoms. Embracing the mind-body connection isn't just feel-good rhetoric; it's about leveraging the profound impacts that mental fortitude, self-belief, and resilience can have on our overall well-being. Whether it's through the silent affirmations that greet us in the mirror or the visualization techniques that cast our challenges in a more manageable light, these tools are not just accessories to our menopause strategy, they are essential components. They are the silent architects of our strength, sculpting the grace with which we adapt and thrive. As we dive deeper, we'll explore how installing these practices into your daily regime can ground you in positivity and how cultivating this empowering outlook is as vital as any supplement or therapy you engage with.

Developing a Positive Outlook

Transitioning into a new phase of life is like navigating uncharted waters – it requires an open heart, courage, and, above all, a positive outlook. In the tumultuous sea of hormonal changes, a mindset that embraces optimism can be your anchor. Let's illuminate ways to cultivate such an outlook, ensuring that menopause becomes an enriching period rather than a disheartening one. Remember, what's happening in your body isn't a setback; it's a natural progression, and your attitude can make all the difference in experiencing it with grace and vitality.

Firstly, understand that positivity isn't about wearing rose-color glasses all the time. Acknowledge the challenges and the frustrations that come with menopause without letting them define your entire experience. Think about those hot flashes as reminders of the incredible power of your body, adapting and signaling in its unique language. When you start interpreting your body's messages more gently and positively, the physical experiences can take on a different, less daunting quality. It's about framing – viewing this time as a season of renewal, not just of loss.

Next, surrounding yourself with laughter, joy, and activities that light up your soul is crucial. Laughter can be a surprisingly potent medicine. Whether it's a giggly lunch with friends, a quirky sitcom, or a hilarious book, incorporating laughter into your day-to-day life can lift your spirits. More importantly, it can shift your focus from the symptoms you're enduring to the moments of joy you're experiencing. Plus, engaging in hobbies or activities that nurture your spirit can replenish your energy and give you a sense of accomplishment and purpose.

It's also super beneficial to start each day with intention. Begin with a few positive affirmations about your strength and resilience. Try keeping a gratitude journal – write down a couple of things you're thankful for each morning, and see how such a simple act can reshape your outlook. Regularly recognizing the abundance in your life, rather than its perceived shortages, turns the mind into an ally that fuels your journey through menopause with hope, instead of a critic that weighs you down with doubt.

Last but not least, don't isolate yourself. A heart-to-heart talk with someone who gets it can do wonders. Connect with others undergoing similar transitions by joining support groups or forums. Sharing stories and solutions helps forge a collective strength that not only supports you but also allows you to be a beacon for someone else. A sturdy network of friends, loved ones, or fellow voyagers on this journey can help you maintain a positive outlook and affirm that you're not alone in this. Embracing menopause as a community can transform this time into a shared adventure, rather than a solitary trial.

Garnering a positive outlook during menopause is like tending a garden; it needs attention, nurturing, and patience. Positivity blooms from deliberate steps - recognizing your strengths, seeking joy, practicing gratitude, connecting with others, and reaffirming the beauty in this natural shift. By fostering a healthy mindset, you're not merely enduring menopause; you're thriving through it, and setting the stage for a post-menopausal life filled with wellness and wonder.

Mind-Body Connection and Menopause

The journey through menopause can feel like a rollercoaster for both the body and psyche, but embracing the profound connection between the two can transform this transition into a path of self-discovery and empowerment. It's essential to recognize that the mind's tapestry is intricately woven with the physical fluctuations of menopause; thoughts and attitudes hold power in shaping the experience of symptoms. Envision being in the driver's seat, with mindfulness as your GPS, guiding you to navigate mood swings and hot flashes with a sense of control and grace. Integrating meditation, deep-breathing exercises, or yoga into your routine isn't just a dalliance in relaxation; these are acts of reclaiming your equilibrium, aligning the mental and somatic domains in harmonious conversation. Your body listens to the stories your mind tells, so let's author a narrative of resilience and well-being, knowing that the mindset you cultivate can influence your menopausal voyage as much as any supplement or workout. Celebrate this interplay, knowing you're nurturing not just a symptom, but the whole magnificent garden that is you.

Harnessing the Power of Belief can be a transformative approach to navigating menopause, where the waves of change threaten to unsettle the familiar shores we've walked through much of womanhood. It's time to embrace the mind's profound influence on the body. When we talk about belief, we aren't diving into magical thinking; instead, we're recognizing the science-backed tenet that the mind-body connection is mighty – especially throughout menopause.

Your inner dialogue has the power to shape your day-to-day life, inclusive of how you experience the symptoms and challenges of menopause. Cognitive reframing can help transform how you perceive hot flashes, night sweats, and mood swings. A combative stance might heighten frustration, but an acceptance-based strategy could soften your reaction, transforming each symptom into an opportunity for mindfulness and gratitude for your body's resilience. It's not trivializing the experience; it's giving you back control.

Empowering beliefs can also catalyze the effectiveness of natural therapies. When combined with a healthy dose of skepticism and a commitment to personal well-being, believing in your chosen path of holistic health can enhance the impact of dietary shifts, targeted exercises, or relaxation practices. A balanced perspective is key–being both open-minded about natural treatment options and also aware of their limitations, grounding your beliefs in research and personal fit.

Evoking change with belief isn't instant; it's a practice. Integrating positive beliefs into your daily routine through affirmations or visualization might feel awkward at first, yet, over time, they'll become part of the fabric of your being. Picture your beliefs as a garden – with consistent care and attention, they can flourish and transform the landscape of your menopause experience.

Remember, your beliefs set the stage for your actions. Believing that you can navigate this transition with strength and grace encourages proactive measures for self-care, opens up avenues for learning, and fosters resilience. This internal groundwork lays a strong foundation for blending hormone therapy with natural remedies, crafting a menopause strategy as unique as you are. Harness the inherent power of your belief, and watch as it becomes one of the most potent tools in your holistic health arsenal.

Using Visualization and Affirmations

Embarking on the menopause journey, we've dissected hormone therapy, turned every nutritional leaf, and touched on the importance of physical activity. Now, let's dive into the sea of the mind, where visualization and affirmations become life rafts amidst the waves of change. Visualization is not just a daydream; it's a deliberate and powerful technique that can shape our perception, attitude, and ultimately, our health. Envision the best version of yourself: confident, healthy, radiating calm amidst menopause's storms. This imagery can be the compass that guides you through daily challenges, reinforcing your resilience and strength.

Similarly, affirmations are like seeds planted in the fertile ground of our subconscious. They germinate powerful beliefs that blossom into reality. Whisper words of encouragement to yourself - "I am strong," "I navigate menopause with ease," or "I am in tune with my body." Express these affirmations with conviction, and watch as they fortify your spirit, helping to quell hot flashes of doubt, and bloom into a garden of positivity. Combine these affirmations with visualization, and you've got a dynamic duo that can reset your emotional thermostat.

How can you practice these techniques effectively? Start by anchoring your visualizations in the present moment, as if you're already living the life you desire. The mind often can't differentiate between what's real and what's vividly imagined. Similarly, affirm affirmations out loud, in front of a mirror, infusing them with passion and belief. Do this daily - consistency waters these mental seeds, helping you build a landscape that's more harmonious with your menopause adventure.

Remember, menopause might sometimes feel like a mapless endeavor, but with visualization and affirmations, you're sketching the map yourself. These practices provide comfort and direction when physical symptoms and emotional turbulences want to take the wheel. They are the undercurrent pushing you gently towards a shore of tranquility and balance, reminding you that you have the power to shape your experience.

As we close this section, take with you the understanding that your mind is an ally, a tool at your disposal to craft your experience of menopause. By harnessing the power of visualization and affirmations, you're not just passively awaiting change; you're actively creating it. Let these practices be the lighthouse guiding you to the well-being you deserve. They are instruments for not just surviving this transformation, but thriving through it.

Chapter 13:
Preparing for Post-Menopause

As we close the chapter on menopause, it's time to turn the page, ladies, and embrace the incredible journey that lies ahead in post-menopause. Consider this transition not as an end but as a vibrant new beginning—a time to nurture your body and soul with long-term health strategies, tailored to your unique journey into a life beyond the hormones' wild ride. You've weathered the storm of hot flashes, navigated the ebbs and flows of emotional tides, and now, you're ready to embark on an empowering voyage of sustained wellness. Let's cultivate that inner garden of health by delving into preventative care that keeps your heart strong, bones fortified, and energy replenished. It's about rekindling passions, fostering connections that enrich your spirit, and creating a legacy that sparkles with the wisdom of your years. In post-menopause, you'll be writing a story where every chapter celebrates the essence of who you've become—a life marked not just by the years, but the life in your years.

Long-Term Health Strategies

As you navigate through the winding path of menopause and step boldly into the postmenopausal phase of life, it's vital to focus on long-term health strategies that will sustain and nourish you. Think of it as cultivating a lush garden — it requires ongoing attention and care. A vital aspect of this is bone health; as estrogen levels decline, your risk of osteoporosis rises. A balanced diet rich in calcium and vitamin D, weight-bearing exercises, and perhaps even a chat with your doctor about medication can make a world of difference. It's about embracing these habits not just as a must-do but as a loving nod to your future self.

Let's talk heart health – your heart has been with you through thick and thin, and it's going to need your consideration even more now. As estrogen takes a bow, your risk for cardiovascular issues can sneak up. But fear not, incorporating heart-healthy foods that are low in saturated fats and cholesterol, and saying hello to regular physical activity, can keep your ticker humming along. And if you smoke, consider this a friend nudging you-with kindness and support-to leave that habit by the wayside. Remember, protecting your heart is really about giving yourself a hug from the inside.

Then there's the buzz around the brain – yep, your cognitive health is pivotal, and it loves a good workout too. Mental exercises, puzzles, continuous learning, and even social interaction can keep your neurons firing and your wit as sharp as ever. It's about weaving a tapestry of intellectual stimulation throughout your daily life —be it through a book club, language class, or simply a spirited debate with friends.

Now, while focusing on the physical is significant, let's not overlook the emotional landscape. Tending to your mental health by fostering strong relationships, indulging in your passions, and possibly seeking guidance from a therapist can keep the blues at bay. It's about crafting an emotional toolkit that works for you, that helps you navigate the waters of life with resilience and joy. And laughter, never underestimate the power of laughter—it's like a warm balm for the soul.

In essence, your post-menopausal years are a time to shine, with the wisdom of experience and the freedom that comes with it. It's not just about surviving; it's about thriving, flourishing, and savoring every moment. These long-term health strategies aren't just items on a checklist; they are your stepping stones to a vibrant, fulfilling life. So carry forward with intention and gusto, knowing that every small step you take is a leap towards a jubilant and healthy future.

Embracing a New Phase of Life

Transitioning into post-menopause is like venturing into a fresh chapter, where embracing change becomes the mantra for a vibrant future. It's not just about saying bye to the tampons and hello to a newfound freedom; it's a powerful period of self-reinvention and boundless opportunities. You've navigated the waves of hormonal ebbs and flows and now it's time to set sail on calm seas, finding strength in the stability that lies ahead. With hot flashes and night sweats becoming tales of the past, there's an invigorating space to fill with activities and passions that resonate with your true self. Consider this: the wisdom and experience you've gleaned through the menopause journey are your badges of honor, and this is your moment to shine without the shadow of a symptom tracker. Let's cherish this transition, taking care not to wish away these moments but to weave them into the rich tapestry of life. Reclaim your energy and focus on what makes you thrive—whether it's delving into hobbies that were on hold, investing in relationships, or simply enjoying a serene cup of tea without the sudden heatwave. Post-menopause isn't an end, it's a celebration of resilience and a testament to your body's natural grace—it's time to embrace all its promise with open arms and a courageous heart.

Maintaining Wellness Beyond Menopause means acknowledging that while one significant phase of your life has transitioned, another vibrant, active chapter is just beginning. Think of your post-menopausal years as a canvas, and wellness as your palette; you have the power to create a masterpiece. It's a time when you can tune into your body's rhythms and needs without the ebb and flow of the menstrual cycle. Instead of viewing menopause as a finale, consider it an intermission, after which you can re-enter life's theater with vitality and a renewed focus on holistic health.

During these years, consistency is key in your wellness routine. In synergy with prescribed hormone therapy, incorporating natural practices into your daily life can continue to play a significant role in how you feel. Lean into a diet rich in phytoestrogens, which can help maintain a natural hormonal balance. Prioritize nutrients dense in antioxidants and ensure you're getting enough calcium and vitamin D, as these are crucial for bone health, which can be affected after menopause. Keep moving with an exercise regimen that suits your pace - be it yoga, walking, or dance - and your bones, heart, and muscles will thank you.

But let's not overlook the power of the mind. Positive thinking, mindfulness, and a strong support network are invaluable. They nourish the soul just like a balanced diet nourishes the body. Practice self-compassion and recognize the strength it has taken to get to this chapter. Strengthen your connections with friends, family, and groups who uplift you and understand the journey you're on. Share your experiences and draw on the collective wisdom of those who walk alongside you. Beyond lifestyle tweaks, it's about crafting a holistic mindset because embracing change and maintaining wellness isn't just about what you do—it's about how you think, react, and persevere on this journey of post-menopausal self-discovery.

Legacy and Empowerment

As you embrace the new phase of life that comes after menopause, it's time to reflect on the legacy you'd like to leave and the ways you can empower yourself and others. Menopause isn't an ending; it's a gateway to a period rich with potential for growth and self-discovery. Think about the wisdom you've accumulated—the struggles you've overcome—and how you can share that with the world. Maybe it's through mentoring, launching a new project, or simply being a vocal advocate for women's health.

Empowerment during this stage is about taking control of your health and happiness. It's realizing that you have the autonomy to make choices that align with your desires and needs. Align your menopause strategy by pursuing activities that elevate your well-being and connect you with a community. Consider joining or forming a group focused on holistic menopause care, where members can exchange natural remedies, support each other through changes, and celebrate milestones together.

Your embodiment of strength and resilience can radically change perceptions of aging and menopause. It's vital to champion the narrative that women in post-menopause are pillars of knowledge and power, not just in their circles but in society at large. Write, speak, and live your truth. You're not just passing through menopause; you're setting a precedent for future generations who will look to your experience as a beacon of enlightenment and encouragement.

Self-empowerment also comes from nurturing your aspirations and interests that may have been on hold. Maybe you have a passion that took a backseat during other life phases. Now's the time to reignite that spark. Whether it's art, science, business, or activism, pursuing these avenues can become part of the legacy you create. They serve as a testament to the fact that growth and fulfillment are not confined to the so-called 'youthful' years.

Lastly, remember the importance of self-compassion and kindness. These are the cornerstone of empowerment. As you glide through post-menopause, your body and mind will continue to evolve. Approach every change with grace and patience, knowing that with each day, you're cultivating a legacy of empowerment not just for yourself but for all women navigating this natural and transformative journey.

Conclusion

As we reach the end of our journey together, it's time to reflect on the wisdom shared, the strategies discussed, and the sense of empowerment you've hopefully gained. Menopause may have felt like an unsure voyage at times, but through embracing a holistic health strategy that combines hormone therapy with natural practices, we can navigate these waters with grace and vitality. The symphony of your body's needs is unique, and tuning into that music with a personalized approach can make all the difference. People across the world are captivated by the idea of living vibrantly through all stages of life - and you are no different. You have the power to turn the tide in favor of a fulfilling menopause transition.

Remember, integrating hormone therapy with an array of natural remedies isn't about choosing sides; it's about creating harmony within your body. Diet, exercise, stress management, sleep hygiene, and the consideration of alternative therapies form an orchestra of options that can play in sync with medical treatments. By keeping a close eye on how your body and mind respond, adjusting your strategy, and working closely with healthcare providers, you'll find the right rhythm for your menopause symphony.

Sexual health, skincare, and nurturing supportive environments are just as crucial in the grand design of your menopause strategy. They are not solitary notes but are woven into the fabric of your overall well-being. Maintaining open communication with your partner, understanding the hormonal impacts on your skin and hair, and fostering social connections ensure you live this chapter of life as fully as any other.

As we've explored the holistic realm of menopause management, it's clear that mindset plays a pivotal role. A positive outlook, a belief in your body's resilience, and the power of visualization open up a world of potential for health and happiness. Embrace this change with both arms, knowing it's another phase of growth and discovery. Hold on to the fact that beyond the horizon of menopause is a vast sea of opportunity - post-menopause - where you can continue to thrive, preserve wellness, and leave a legacy of empowerment for others following in your wake.

In closing, this is not an end but a beginning. It's the start of you taking charge, with the tools and knowledge you now possess, to live every day with intention and joy. The narrative of menopause is yours to write, and each page can be filled with strength, wisdom, and holistic health. Go forth with confidence, knowing that each step you take is part of a broader, more beautiful journey.

Appendix A:
Appendix

As we've navigated the rich tapestry of menopause, from demystifying its symptoms to embracing a holistic lifestyle that includes both hormone therapy and natural remedies, it's time to offer you a collection of resources that will keep you supported on your journey. We believe knowledge is not just power—it's peace of mind, a comforter, and a pathfinder all rolled into one.

A. Resources for Further Reading

Embarking on this journey towards a comprehensive approach to menopause demands resources that are both reliable and empowering. To quench your thirst for knowledge and to find solace in the experiences of others, we've gathered a list of resources where you can dive deeper into various topics related to menopause. The books, websites, and articles we suggest here offer a wealth of information and inspiration, encouraging you to learn and grow with every page you turn or click you make.

Whether you're looking to expand your understanding of hormone replacement therapy's nuances or explore the breadth of natural practices out there, we've got you covered. Our selection includes works from esteemed professionals who have dedicated their careers to women's health, as well as personal narratives that resonate with the heart and soul of the matter. And because menopause touches upon so many aspects of life, from intimacy to skin care, we've made sure to cover a spectrum that's as broad and diverse as the experiences of women going through this natural phase.

B. Symptom Tracker and Journal Prompts

Self-awareness is key in managing menopause effectively. With that in mind, we're providing you with tools to track your symptoms and reflect on your feelings through carefully designed journal prompts. These resources aim to help you connect the dots between your lifestyle choices and the shifts in your symptoms, offering insights into what works best for you. Tracking and journaling foster a spirit of self-care that's proactive, mindful, and deeply personal—they're acts of love you dedicate to yourself daily.

The symptom tracker will help you monitor changes, identify triggers, and note patterns. This can be incredibly useful when discussing treatments with your healthcare provider or when deciding to try new natural remedies. The journal prompts, on the other hand, are here to support your emotional well-being, inviting introspection and providing clarity amidst the flux of change. They'll encourage you to pause, breathe, and recalibrate, ensuring that your journey through menopause is as reflective as it is informed.

As your path unfolds, remember that the power lies within you. With each step, you are crafting a life that's rich in well-being, bolstered by knowledge, and surrounded by a community of support. Embrace this transition with grace, strength, and the joy of knowing that you're wholly capable of thriving through menopause and beyond.

C. Resources for Further Reading

As we close the book on our comprehensive journey through menopause, you might find yourself curious about diving even deeper into some topics. There's a world of information waiting for you to explore, and we've sifted through the wilderness of words to give you a trail to follow. Whether you're looking to expand your knowledge on hormone therapy alternatives, seeking delicious recipes that balance hormones, or wanting inspiration for mindfulness techniques, we've got your back. Our carefully curated reading list is packed with thought-provoking, comforting, and progressive reads that embrace the power and potential of menopause. Let these books be companions in your ongoing journey.

When it comes to nutrition, the information out there can be overwhelming. But fear not, we've found some fantastic books that will guide you through the essentials of eating for hormonal balance with ease. They're not just about diets, they're about enjoying food in a way that nurtures your body and soul. Look for books that celebrate natural ingredients and come with recipes that are as easy to execute as they are beneficial. Some even come with meal plans tailored to alleviate specific menopausal symptoms, making the transition smoother and tastier.

If you've been inspired by our chapters on physical wellbeing, we recommend books that will take you further into the world of exercise, specifically focusing on the needs of your body during menopause. These books should offer practical advice on everything from yoga to strength training—aligning with your body's changing needs. Plus, they'll often come with step-by-step guides, providing clear images and directions to ensure your form is perfect and your mind is as engaged as your muscles.

Mindfulness and relaxation are not just passing trends; they are essential tools for managing stress and enhancing sleep quality, especially during menopause. That's why we'll point you towards books filled with strategies to quiet your mind and soothe your spirit. Whether it's through guided meditations, breathing techniques, or cognitive resets, these reads aim to turn your moments of tranquility into powerful rituals that rejuvenate your mental and emotional well-being.

And let's not overlook the incredibly rich realm of herbal remedies and alternative therapies that exist alongside hormone therapy. For those of you intrigued by the potential of plants and herbal wisdom, we've got some great titles to suggest. These books delve deep into the science and tradition of herbal medicine, providing practical advice on how to integrate these remedies into your daily life safely and effectively.

Your journey doesn't stop with the last page of this book—consider it a beginning. With each further reading suggestion, we hope you'll feel more empowered, enlightened, and invested in your menopausal voyage. Embrace these resources, and let your curiosity lead you to newfound strength and understanding of your body's transformation.

D. Symptom Tracker and Journal Prompts

If you're like many women going through this transition, you might find that your menopause journey is as unique as you are. One day you might be all pep and productivity, and the next, fatigue could set in like an unwelcome houseguest. It can be a rollercoaster - but having a way to track your symptoms and reflections can be empowering. It's not just about jotting down what you're experiencing; it's about uncovering patterns, recognizing triggers, and appreciating the nuances of your body's messages.

A symptom tracker does more than remind you of the hot flashes or the occasional mood swing. It's a tool that brings clarity, revealing the ebb and flow of your body's conversation with you. By tracking your symptoms with diligence and honesty, you're effectively saying, "Okay, body, I'm listening—let's figure this out together." You'll start noticing if certain foods, activities, or even times of day are nudging those symptoms in one direction or another, equipping you with the insights to make tweaks to your lifestyle or treatment plan.

Journal prompts, on the other hand, are your secret superpower. They beckon you to dig deeper, beyond the surface-level symptoms. Each prompt is an invitation to explore more than what's happening, but how you're truly feeling about it. Let's face it—menopause isn't always going to be front-page news or the hot topic at your weekly coffee catch-up. But in your journal? You're the editor-in-chief, and every thought, fear, victory, and giggle is headline-worthy. Journaling morphs those thoughts swirling around your head into a roadmap for self-discovery and healing.

Integrating these practices can be a game-changer. Start by setting aside a few moments each day—maybe that's right after your morning routine or before the lights go out at night. Use your tracker to log the physical stuff, the nuts and bolts of your body's workings. Then take a breath and dive into a journal prompt. One day might call for reflection on gratitude and the next on how shifts in your body image are impacting your sense of self. These prompts don't need to have any rules—just let the pen flow and see where it takes you. That way, you're not just living through menopause; you're actively participating in it, harnessing its insights to fuel your journey forward.

Remember, there's no 'right' way to navigate this chapter of your life, but having a personalized map sure can help. The symphony of your bodily changes has a rhythm you can learn, and with your journal as your compass, you might just find yourself dancing along. So let's do this; let's tap into that wellspring of inner knowledge, because you've got more wisdom in you than you might realize, and it's just waiting to spill out onto those pages.

E. Glossary of Terms

As we weave together the many threads of information that create a colorful tapestry of menopausal understanding, it's essential to have a clear grasp on the terminology we're using. Sometimes, the medical jargon can be as puzzling as a hot flash in winter. So, let's clear the fog with some down-to-earth explanations of the terms you'll often come across on this journey.

Bioidentical Hormones

These are hormones that are chemically identical to those your body naturally produces. They're often suggested as a more "natural" approach to hormone therapy, but it's important to know that 'natural' doesn't always mean 'safer' or 'better.'

Cognitive Behavioral Therapy (CBT)

This is a type of psychotherapy that helps you manage problems by changing the way you think and behave. It's particularly useful if you're dealing with mood swings or anxiety during menopause. What's happening in your mind can have a huge impact on how you feel physically.

Endocrine System

Think of this as your body's hormone headquarters. It's a collection of glands that produce and release hormones which regulate a whole host of bodily functions - including your menstrual cycle.

Estrogen

One of the key hormonal players in the female body, estrogen, takes a bow as you progress through menopause. Its levels decrease, which can lead to various symptoms. It's not just about hot flashes; it's deeply involved in bone health, brain function, and the health of your heart.

Homeopathy

A form of alternative medicine founded on the idea that the body can heal itself. It uses tiny amounts of natural substances like plants and minerals. While some swear by its gentle approach, it's always good to consult with your health provider to see if it fits into your wellness puzzle.

Libido

This is the fancy term for your sex drive. You might find it doing the cha-cha on a rollercoaster during menopause. It can be a touchy subject, but it's normal to experience changes in your desire – and there are ways to get your groove back!

Mindfulness

This practice is all about living in the 'right now'. By focusing your awareness on the present moment, while calmly acknowledging and accepting your feelings, it can be an incredible tool to manage stress and promote inner peace. Menopause can be a wild ride, but a mindful approach can keep you grounded.

Phytoestrogens

Pull these plant-based compounds into your dietary dance. They can mimic or modulate estrogen in your body, and they're found in foods like soy – ever versatile, a bit like your wardrobe should be during hot flash season!

Progesterone

Another hormone that tapers off as you march towards menopause. It works in concert with estrogen and plays a key role during your menstrual cycle and in maintaining pregnancies.

Sleep Hygiene

Not about scrubbing your sheets every night, but rather the habits that help you score consistent, quality Z's. Considering sleep can become as elusive as a calm house during a family reunion, sleep hygiene is critical.

It's a lot to digest, and some days you might feel like you're cramming for a menopausal midterm. But understanding these terms can empower you to make informed decisions about your journey through menopause. Remember, each experience is as unique as you, and armed with knowledge, you're already on the path to thriving during this transformative stage of life.

F. Hormone Therapy and Natural Remedies FAQ

It's likely that you've got a mix of curiosity and apprehension swirling around hormone therapy and natural remedies. You're not alone. These are vital tools for navigating menopause, and it sure can feel like you need a guidebook. Well, consider this section to be just that. Here, we'll chat about some of the most pressing questions that come up when merging these two worlds. Think of it as having a heart-to-heart over coffee with your go-to menopause guru.

First up, it's natural to wonder if you can mix hormone therapy with herbal supplements. The short answer is: it depends. Every body is unique, and so is every remedy. Some herbs might interact with hormones in ways that crank up the effectiveness or dial it down. It's crucial to loop in a healthcare provider who's savvy about both prescription meds and nature's offerings. They'll help ensure you're pairing them up safely and effectively, just like finding the perfect blend for your morning smoothie.

Looking at the flip side, you might ponder if natural remedies alone can take the edge off those pesky hot flashes and mood swings. For some, the answer is a resounding "yes," and for others, it's a mix of "sort of" and "I need a bit more help here." Remember, there's no one-size-fits-all. Plants and lifestyle tweaks have potent powers, but it's about finding the right concoction for you. So don't be shy about experimenting with various herbs, foods, and activities that sing to your particular body's needs.

How will you know if your hormone therapy or natural remedy cocktail is working? Tune into your body. It's a sophisticated sensor that can communicate in subtle nudges or loud alarms. Keep track of what's going on—a little journaling goes a long way. See how you feel as you go about your day, check your sleep quality, and notice if you're dancing through hot flashes or gritting your teeth. And remember, this isn't a "set it and forget it" kind of deal; adjustments may be necessary along the journey.

Lastly, the ever-lingering question of side effects—because let's face it, nobody signs up for those. Whether you're taking hormone therapy, sipping herbal teas, or embracing lifestyle changes, side effects can be part of the package. But the trick lies in communication and being proactive. Keep your healthcare team in the loop with what you're experiencing. Together, you'll be able to navigate these waters, adjusting your sails as needed to ensure the smoothest sail possible through menopause.

Remember, this journey through menopause is yours—and it's unique. Just like you. So, pull together your personal mix of modern medicine, age-old plant wisdom, and lifestyle tweaks. It can take a bit of trial and error, but that's okay. You're crafting a menopause strategy that's as tailor-made for you as your favorite playlist. Let's get you feeling like you've got this because, believe it or not—you absolutely do.

www.ingramcontent.com/pod-product-compliance
Lightning Source LLC
Chambersburg PA
CBHW020334290526
45785CB00005B/2004